T0100137

Pocket Prescriber Pulmonary Medicine

Pocket Prescriber Pulmonary Medicine

Craig Batista
Consultant in Respiratory Medicine
Guy's and St Thomas' NHS Foundation Trust
London, UK

Donald RJ Singer
President, Fellowship of Postgraduate Medicine, UK

Peter J Barnes
Margaret Turner-Warwick Professor of Medicine
National Heart and Lung Institute
and
Honorary Consultant Physician
Royal Brompton Hospital
London, UK

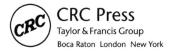

CRC Press
Taylor & Francis Group
Boca Raton London New York

CRC Press is an imprint of the
Taylor & Francis Group, an **informa** business

First edition published 2024
by CRC Press
6000 Broken Sound Parkway NW, Suite 300, Boca Raton, FL 33487-2742

and by CRC Press
2 Park Square, Milton Park, Abingdon, Oxon, OX14 4RN

CRC Press is an imprint of Taylor & Francis Group, LLC

ISBN: 9781498744409 (pbk)
ISBN: 9781315151816 (ebk)

DOI: 10.1201/9781315151816

Typeset in Sabon LT Std
by KnowledgeWorks Global Ltd.

CONTENTS

FOREWORD

This much needed new edition of the *Pocket Prescriber Pulmonary Medicine* is very timely in view of the many changes in approach and the many new drugs that have been introduced for respiratory diseases in recent years. The succinct format of the book makes it extremely valuable to busy clinicians who need to obtain information rapidly and easily. The treatment strategy and indications for particular drugs for each respiratory disease is clearly set out, providing a rationale for prescribing each therapy. This compact book covers airway diseases, interstitial lung diseases, respiratory infections (including tuberculosis), pulmonary hypertension, lung cancer, transplantation and palliative care. The text is bang up to date and includes the use of inhaled corticosteroids + formoterol inhalers as relievers in asthma as well as the indications for the new biological therapies introduced for severe eosinophilic asthma. The many combination inhalers available for COPD patients that combine long-acting bronchodilators, as well as triple inhalers are included. There is a very useful section on how to deliver different types of therapy, with a valuable section on the many different inhaler devices and how they should be used. There is also a section on the use of drugs in respiratory emergencies. This pocketbook provides an enormous amount of current information on prescribing therapies for the whole range of respiratory diseases in a compact and easily accessible format. It also provides key information about adverse effects and drug interactions. This book will of great value to the busy respiratory clinician, whether in a hospital setting or in private and general practice at all levels, but will be particularly useful for doctors in training who need to make rapid decisions about management.

Professor Peter Barnes
FRS, FMedSci
National Heart and Lung Institute,
Imperial College London

ACKNOWLEDGEMENTS

I want to thank you to all my teachers, mentors and colleagues from whom I have learnt, and continue to learn, so much. Especially to Tim Nicholson and the late Donald Singer for masterminding this latest edition in the pocket prescriber series, and for all their hard work and invaluable guidance along the way. It was an absolute pleasure working with both of you. Special thanks must also go to respiratory pharmacists Elaine Bowman and Mami Harrison for their review of the manuscript.

I wish to dedicate this book to my ever-patient wife Anitha and my little man Luka. I also wish to pay a special tribute to Donald who was such a kind, patient and learned mentor. He is sorely missed by all after his untimely passing.

The information in this book has been collected from many sources, including manufacturer's information sheets ('SPCs' – Summary of Product Characteristics sheets), the British National Formulary (BNF), national and international guidelines, as well as numerous pharmacology and general medical books, journals and papers. Where information is not consistent between these sources, that from the SPCs has generally been taken as definitive.

Craig Batista
April 2023

STANDARD LAYOUT OF DRUGS

DRUG/TRADE NAME

Class/action: More information is given for generic forms, especially for the original and most commonly used drug(s) of each class.

Use: use^x (correlating to dose as follows).

CI: contraindications; **L** (liver failure), **R** (renal failure), **H** (heart failure), **P** (pregnancy), **B** (breastfeeding). *Allergy to active drug or any excipients (other substances in the preparation) assumed too obvious to mention.*

Caution: **L** (liver failure), **R** (renal failure), **H** (heart failure), **P** (pregnancy), **B** (breastfeeding), **E** (elderly patients). If a contraindication is given for a drug, it is assumed too obvious to mention that a caution is also inherently implied.

SE: side effects; listed in order of frequency encountered. Common/important side effects set in **bold**.

Warn: information to give to patients before starting drug.

Monitor: parameters that need to be monitored during treatment.

Interactions: included only if very common or potentially serious; ↑/↓P450 (induces/inhibits cytochrome P450 metabolism), **W+** (increases effect of warfarin), **W–** (decreases effect of warfarin).

Dose: dose^x (for use^x as previously mentioned). *NB: Doses are for adults only.*

Important points highlighted at end of drug entries.

Use/dose[NICE]: National Institute for Health and Care Excellence (NICE) guidelines exist for the drug (basics often in the *British National Formulary* [BNF] – see https://www.nice.org.uk for full details).

Dose[BNF/SPC]: dose regimen complicated; please refer to BNF and/or SPC (Summary of Product Characteristics sheet; the manufacturer's information sheet enclosed with drug packaging – can also be viewed at or downloaded from https://www.emc.medicines.org.uk. **Asterisks (*)** and **daggers (†)** denote links between information within local text. Other sources:

BAP	Guidance from the British Association for Psychopharmacology
MPG	*The Maudsley Prescribing Guidelines in Psychiatry*, 13E
SIGN	Scottish Intercollegiate Guidelines Network
UKTIS	UK Teratology Information Service
UKDILAS	UK Drugs in Lactation Advisory Service
NEPTUNE	Novel Psychoactive Treatment: UK Network

Only relevant sections are included for each drug. **Trade names** (in **solid grey** font) are given only if found regularly on drug charts or if non-proprietary (generic, non-trade-name) drug does not yet exist.

KEY

- ☠ Potential dangers highlighted with skull and crossbones
- ▼ New drug or new indication under intense surveillance by the Committee on Safety of Medicines (CSM): *important to report all suspected drug reactions via Yellow Card Scheme* (accurate as going to press: from May 2019 European Medicines Agency list)
- ☺ *Good for:* reasons to give a certain drug when choice exists
- ☹ *Bad for:* reasons to not give a certain drug when choice exists
- ⇒ Causes/goes to
- ∴ Therefore
- Δ Change/disturbance
- Ψ Psychiatric
- ↑ Increase/high
- ↓ Decrease/low
- ✖ Respiratory Failure

↑/↓ electrolytes refer to serum levels, unless stated otherwise.

DOSES

Od	once daily	Nocte	at night
Bd	twice daily	Mane	in the morning
Tds	three times daily	Prn	as required
Qds	four times daily	Stat	at once

ROUTES

Im	Intramuscular	po	oral
Inh	Inhaled	pr	rectal
Iv	Intravenous	sc	subcutaneous
Ivi	intravenous infusion	top	topical
Neb	via nebuliser	sl	sublingual

Routes are presumed po, unless stated otherwise.

LIST OF ABBREVIATIONS

5-ASA	5-aminosalicylic acid
5-HT	5-hydroxytryptamine (= serotonin)
A&E	accident & emergency
AAC	antibiotic-associated colitis
Ab	antibody
abdo	abdomen/abdominal
ABG	arterial blood gases
ABPM	ambulatory blood pressure monitoring
ACC	American College of Cardiology
ACCP	American College of Chest Physicians
ACE-i	angiotensin-converting enzyme (ACE) inhibitor
ACh	acetylcholine
ACS	acute coronary syndrome
ADP	adenosine diphosphate
AF	atrial fibrillation
Ag	antigen
AHA	American Heart Association
AKI	acute kidney injury
ALL	acute lymphoblastic leukaemia
ALP	alkaline phosphatase
ALS	Adult Life Support (algorithms of the European Resuscitation Council)
ALT	alanine (-amino) transferase
AMI	acute myocardial infarction
AMTS	abbreviated mental test score (same as MTS)
ANA	anti-nuclear antigen
APTT	activated partial thromboplastin time
ARB	angiotensin receptor blocker
ARDS	adult respiratory distress syndrome
AS	aortic stenosis
ASAP	as soon as possible
assoc	associated
AST	aspartate transaminase
AV	arteriovenous

AVM	arteriovenous malformation
AVN	atrioventricular node
AZT	zidovudine
BAP	British Association for Psychopharmacology
BBB	bundle branch block
BCSH	British Committee for Standards in Haematology
BCT	broad complex tachycardia
Bd	bis in die
BF	blood flow
BG	serum blood glucose in mmol/L; *see also* CBG (capillary blood glucose)
BHS	British Hypertension Society
BIH	benign intracranial hypertension
BIPAP	bilevel/biphasic positive airway pressure
BM	bone marrow (*NB:* BM is often used, confusingly, to signify finger-prick glucose; CBG [capillary blood glucose] is used for this purpose in this book)
BMI	body mass index = weight (kg)/height (m)^2
BNF	British National Formulary
BP	blood pressure
BPAD	bipolar affective disorder
BPH	benign prostatic hypertrophy
BTS	British Thoracic Society
Bx	biopsy
C	constipation
Ca	cancer (*NB:* calcium is abbreviated to Ca^{2+})
Ca^{2+}	calcium
CAH	congenital adrenal hyperplasia
CBF	cerebral blood flow
CBG	capillary blood glucose in mmol/L (finger-prick testing) (*NB:* BM is often used to denote this, but this is confusing and less accurate and thus not used in this book)
CCF	congestive cardiac failure
CCU	coronary care unit

CE	cystic fibrosis
cf	compared with
CI	contraindicated
CK	creatine kinase
CKD	chronic kidney disease
CLL	chronic lymphocytic leukaemia
CML	chronic myelogenous leukaemia
CMV	cytomegalovirus
CNS	central nervous system
CO	cardiac output
COCP	combined oral contraceptive pill
COPD	chronic obstructive pulmonary disease
COX	cyclo-oxygenase
CPR	cardiopulmonary resuscitation
CRF	chronic renal failure
CRP	C-reactive protein
CSF	cerebrospinal fluid
CSM	Committee on Safety of Medicines
CT	computerised tomography
CTO	Community Treatment Order
CVA	cerebrovascular accident
CVD	cardiovascular disease
CVP	central venous pressure
CXR	chest X-ray
D	diarrhoea
$D_{1/2/3 \ldots}$	dopamine receptor subtype$_{1/2/3 \ldots}$
D&V	diarrhoea and vomiting
DA	dopamine
DCT	distal convoluted tubule
dfx	defects
DI	diabetes insipidus
DIC	disseminated intravascular coagulation
DIGAMI	glucose, insulin and potassium intravenous infusion used in acute myocardial infarction
DKA	diabetic ketoacidosis

DM	diabetes mellitus
DMARD	disease-modifying anti-rheumatoid arthritis drug
DOAC	direct oral anticoagulant
DPI	dry powder inhaler
dt	due to
DWI	diffusion-weighted (imaging); specialist magnetic resonance imaging (MRI) mostly used for stroke/ transient ischaemic attack (TIA)
Dx	diagnosis
EØ	eosinophils
e'lyte	electrolyte
EBV	Epstein–Barr virus
ECG	electrocardiogram
ECT	electroconvulsive therapy
EF	ejection fraction
ENT	ear, nose and throat
EPSE	extrapyramidal side effects
ERC	European Resuscitation Council
ESC	European Society of Cardiology
esp	especially
ESR	erythrocyte sedimentation rate
exac	exacerbates
FBC	full blood count
Fe	iron
FFP	fresh frozen plasma
FGA	first generation antipsychotic
FHx	family history
FiO$_2$	inspired O$_2$ concentration
FMF	familial Mediterranean fever
FRIII	fixed rate intravenous insulin infusion
fx	effects
G6PD	glucose-6-phosphate dehydrogenase
GABA	γ-aminobutyric acid
GBS	Guillain–Barré syndrome

GCS	Glasgow Coma Scale
GFR	glomerular filtration rate
GI	gastrointestinal
GIK	glucose, insulin and K^+ infusion
GMC	General Medical Council (of United Kingdom)
GORD	gastro-oesophageal reflux disease
GTN	glyceryl trinitrate
GU	genitourinary
h	hour(s)
H(O)CM	hypertrophic (obstructive) cardiomyopathy
Hb	haemoglobin
HB	heart block
HBPM	home blood pressure monitoring
Hct	haematocrit
HDL	high-density lipoprotein
HF	heart failure
HHS	hyperosmolar hyperglycaemic state
HIV	human immunodeficiency virus
HLA	human leucocyte antigen
HMG-CoA	3-hydroxy-3-methyl-glutaryl coenzyme A
HONK	hyperosmolar non-ketotic state; *see also* HHS (hyperosmolar hyperglycaemic state)
HR	heart rate
hrly	hourly
HSV	herpes simplex virus
Ht	height
HTN	hypertension
HUS	haemolytic uraemic syndrome
Hx	history
IBD	inflammatory bowel disease
IBS	irritable bowel syndrome
IBW	ideal body weight
ICP	intracranial pressure
ICS	inhaled corticosteroid

ICU	intensive care unit
IHD	ischaemic heart disease
IL-2	interleukin-2
im	intramuscular
inc	including
inh	inhaled
INR	international normalised ratio (prothrombin ratio)
IOP	intraocular pressure
ITP	immune/idiopathic thrombocytopenic purpura
ITU	intensive therapy unit
iv	intravenous
IVDU	intravenous drug user
ivi	intravenous infusion
Ix	investigation
JBDS	Joint British Diabetes Societies
JVP	jugular venous pressure
K^+	potassium (serum levels unless stated otherwise)
LØ	lymphocytes
LA	long-acting
LBBB	left bundle branch block
LDL	low-density lipoprotein
LF	liver failure
LFTs	liver function tests
LMWH	low-molecular-weight heparin
LP	lumbar puncture
LVF	left ventricular failure
MØ	macrophages
mane	in morning
MAOI	monoamine oxidase inhibitor
MAP	mean arterial pressure
MCA	middle cerebral artery/Mental Capacity Act
MCV	mean corpuscular volume
metab	metabolised

MG	myasthenia gravis
MHA	Mental Health Act
MHRA	Medicines and Healthcare Products Regulatory Agency (UK)
MI	myocardial infarction
MMF	mycophenolate mofetil
MMSE	Mini-Mental State Examination (scored out of 30*)
MPG	*The Maudsley Prescribing Guidelines in Psychiatry*, 13th Edition
MR	modified release (drug preparation)†
MRI	magnetic resonance imaging
MRSA	methicillin-resistant *Staphylococcus aureus*
MS	multiple sclerosis
MTB	mycobacterium tuberculosis
MTS	(abbreviated) Mental Test Score (scored out of 10*)
MUST	malnutrition universal screening tool
Mx	management
N	nausea
N&V	nausea and vomiting
NØ	neutrophils
NA	noradrenaline (norepinephrine)
Na⁺	sodium (serum levels unless stated otherwise)
NBM	nil by mouth
NCT	narrow complex tachycardia
NDRI	noradrenaline and dopamine reuptake inhibitor
neb	via nebuliser
NEPTUNE	Novel Psychoactive Treatment: UK Network
NGT	nasogastric tube
NH	non-Hodgkin's (lymphoma)
NICE	National Institute for Health and Care Excellence
NIDDM	non-insulin-dependent diabetes mellitus
NIHSS	National (US) Institute of Health Stroke Scale
NIV	non-invasive ventilation
NMDA	N-methyl-D-aspartate
NMJ	neuromuscular junction

NMS	neuroleptic malignant syndrome
NO	nitric oxide
NOAC	novel oral anticoagulant
NPIS	National Poisons Information Service
NSAID	non-steroidal anti-inflammatory drug
NSTEMI	non-ST elevation myocardial infarction
NTM	non-tuberculous mycobacteria
NYHA	New York Heart Association
OCD	obsessive-compulsive disorder
OCP	oral contraceptive pill
OD	overdose (*NB: od = once daily!*)
OGD	oesophagogastroduodenoscopy
OTC	over the counter
p'way(s)	pathway(s)
PAN	polyarteritis nodosa
PBC	primary biliary cirrhosis
PCI	percutaneous coronary intervention (now preferred term for percutaneous transluminal coronary angioplasty [PTCA], which is a subtype of PCI)
PCOS	polycystic ovary syndrome
PCP	*Pneumocystis carinii* pneumonia
PCV	packed cell volume
PD	pharmacodynamics
PDA	patent ductus arteriosus
PE	pulmonary embolism
PEA	pulseless electrical activity
PEF	peak expiratory flow
PEG	percutaneous endoscopic gastrostomy
PG(x)	prostaglandin (receptor subtype *x*)
phaeo	phaeochromocytoma
PHx	past history (of)
PID	pelvic inflammatory disease
PK	pharmacokinetics
PML	progressive multifocal leukoencephalopathy

PMR	polymyalgia rheumatica
po	by mouth (oral)
PO$_4$	phosphate (serum levels, unless stated otherwise)
PPI	proton pump inhibitor
pr	rectal
prep(s)	preparation(s)
prn	as required
PSA	prostate-specific antigen
Pt	platelet(s)
PT	prothrombin time
PTH	parathyroid hormone
PTSD	post-traumatic stress disorder
PU	peptic ulcer
PUO	pyrexia of unknown origin
PVD	peripheral vascular disease
Px	prophylaxis
QT(c)	QT interval (corrected for rate)
RA	rheumatoid arthritis
RAS	renal artery stenosis
RBF	renal blood flow
r/f	refer
RF	renal failure
RID	relative infant dose
RLS	restless legs syndrome
ROSIER	recognition of stroke in emergency room scale for diagnosis of stroke/transient ischaemic attack (TIA)
RR	respiratory rate
RRT	renal replacement therapy
RSV	respiratory syncytial virus
RTI	respiratory tract infection
RV	right ventricle
RVF	right ventricular failure
Rx	treatment

SAH	subarachnoid haemorrhage
SAN	sinoatrial node
SBE	subacute bacterial endocarditis
sc	subcutaneous
SCLE	subacute cutaneous lupus erythematosus
SE(s)	side effect(s)
sec	second(s)
SGA	second generation antipsychotic
SIADH	syndrome of inappropriate antidiuretic hormone
SIGN	Scottish Intercollegiate Guidelines Network
SJS	Stevens–Johnson syndrome
sl	sublingual
SLE	systemic lupus erythematosus
SOA	swelling of ankles
SOB (OE)	shortness of breath (on exertion)
SPC	summary of product characteristic sheet (see page xi, refer to the boxes in 'Standard Layout of Drugs' in 'How to Use This Book')
spp	species
SR	slow/sustained release (drug preparation)
SSRI	selective serotonin reuptake inhibitor
SSS	sick sinus syndrome
STEMI	ST elevation myocardial infarction
supp	suppository
SVT	supraventricular tachycardia
Sx	symptoms
SZ	schizophrenia
$t_{\frac{1}{2}}$	half-life
T_3	triiodothyronine/liothyronine
T_4	thyroxine ($\uparrow$/$\downarrow$ T_4 = hyper-/hypothyroid)
TCA	tricyclic antidepressant
TE	thromboembolism
TEDS	thromboembolism deterrent stockings
TEN	toxic epidermal necrolysis
TFTs	thyroid function tests

TG	triglyceride
TIA	transient ischaemic attack
TIBC	total iron-binding capacity
TIMI score	risk score for unstable angina (UA)/non-ST elevation myocardial infarction (NSTEMI) named after thrombolysis in myocardial infarction (TIMI) trial
TNF	tumour necrosis factor
top	topical
TOXBASE	the primary clinical toxicology database of the National Poisons Information Service
TPMT	thiopurine methyltransferase
TPR	total peripheral resistance
TTA(s)	(drugs) to take away, i.e. prescriptions for inpatients on discharge/leave (aka TTO)
TTO(s)	*see also* TTA
TTP	thrombotic thrombocytopenic purpura
U&Es	urea and electrolytes
UA(P)	unstable angina (pectoris)
UC	ulcerative colitis
UDS	urine drug screen
UKTIS	UK Teratology Information Service
UKDILAS	UK Drugs in Lactation Advisory Service
URTI	upper respiratory tract infection
USS	ultrasound scan
UTI	urinary tract infection
UV	ultraviolet
V	vomiting
VE(s)	ventricular ectopic(s)
VF	ventricular fibrillation
vit	vitamin
VLDL	very-low-density lipoprotein
VRIII	variable rate intravenous insulin infusion
VT	ventricular tachycardia

VTE	venous thromboembolism
VZV	varicella zoster virus (chickenpox/shingles)
w	with
w/in	within
w/o	without
WCC	white cell count
WE	Wernicke's encephalopathy
wk	week
wkly	weekly
WPW	Wolff–Parkinson–White syndrome
Wt	weight
xs	excess
ZE	Zollinger–Ellison syndrome

HOW TO PRESCRIBE SAFELY

Take time/care to ↓ risk to patients (and protect yourself).

Always check the following are correct for all prescriptions: patient, indication and drug, **legible** format (generic name, clarity, handwriting), **identifiable signature**, your contact number), dosage, frequency, time(s) of day, date, duration of treatment, route of administration.

DO

- Make a clear, accurate record in the notes of all medicines prescribed, and indication, written at the time of prescription.
- Complete allergy box and agreed relevant labels and e-alerts.
- Include on all drug charts and TTAs the patient's surname and given name, date of birth, date of admission and consultant (if possible use a printed label for patient details).
- **PRINT** (i.e. use uppercase) all drugs as approved (generic) names, e.g. 'IBUPROFEN' *not* '**nurofen**'.
- State dose, route and frequency, giving strength of solutions/creams.
- Write microgram in full; avoid abbreviations such as mcg or μ.
- Abbreviate the word gram to 'g' (rather than 'gm' which is easily confused with mg).
- Write the word 'units' in full, preceded by a space; abbreviating to 'U' can be misread as zero (a 10-fold error).
- Document weight: guides dosing and GFR calculation.
- Write quantities <1 g in mg (e.g. 400 mg *not* 0.4 g).
- Write quantities <1 mg in micrograms (e.g. 200 micrograms *not* 0.2 mg).
- Write quantities <1 microgram in nanograms (e.g. 500 nanograms *not* 0.5 micrograms).
- Do not use trailing zeroes (10 mg *not* 10.0 mg).
- Precede decimal points with another figure (e.g. 0.8 mL *not* .8 mL), and only use decimals where unavoidable.
- Check and recheck calculations.

- Provide clear additional instructions, e.g. for monitoring, review of antibiotic route and duration, maximum daily/24 h dose for as required drugs.
- Specify solution to be used and duration of any iv infusions/injections.
- Avoid using abbreviated/non-standard drug names.
- Avoid writing 'T' (tablet sign) for non-tablet formulations, e.g. sprays.
- Amend a prescribed drug by drawing a line through it, date and initial this, then rewrite as new prescription.
- Review need for drugs when rewriting a drug chart.
- Check and count number of drugs when rewriting a drug chart.
- Check when prescribing unfamiliar drug(s)/doses or drugs you were familiar with but have not prescribed recently.

IMPORTANT FURTHER ADVICE

1 Make sure choice of drug and dose are right for the patient, their condition and significant comorbidity, with particular attention to age*, gender, ethnicity, renal or liver dysfunction, risk of drug-drug and drug-disease interactions and risks in pregnancy (and those of childbearing age who may become pregnant) and during breastfeeding. Anticipate possible effects of over-the-counter and herbal medicines and lifestyle (e.g. dietary salt and alcohol intake).

   *Although arbitrary, age older than 65 years denotes 'elderly', fx of age can occur earlier/later and are continuous across age spectrum.

2 Common settings where drug problems occur are often predictable if you understand relevant risks, pathology, routes of drug metabolism (liver, P450, renal, etc.) and drug mechanisms of action. Take particular care with
   - Renal or liver disease.
   - Pregnancy/breastfeeding: use safest options (in the United Kingdom consider consulting the UK Teratology Information Service [tel: 0344 8920909]).

- Prescribing or dispensing medicines that could be confused with others (e.g. sound or look similar). See MHRA for examples.
- NSAIDs/bisphosphonates and peptic ulcer disease.
- Asthma and β-blockers.
- Conditions worsened by antimuscarinic drugs (see p. 346, refer 'Cholinoceptors' in 'Side Effect Profiles' in 'Basic Psychopharmacology'): urinary retention/BPH, glaucoma, paralytic ileus.
- Rare conditions where drugs commonly pose risk, e.g. porphyria, myasthenia, G6PD deficiency, phaeo.

3 Always ensure informed consent; agreeing proposed prescriptions with the patient (or carer if patient has authorised their involvement in their care or has lost capacity); explaining proposed benefits, nature and duration of treatment; clarifying concerns; warning of possible, especially severe, adverse effects; highlighting recommended monitoring and review arrangements and stating what the patient should do in the event of a suspected adverse reaction. Only in extreme emergencies can it be justified to have not done this. For drugs with common potentially fatal/severe side effects, document that these risks have been explained to, and accepted by, the patient.

4 See legal advice on eligibility to prescribe and use unlicensed and off-label medicines, checking national guidance (in the UK, see MHRA and GMC guidance).

5 Make sure that you are being objective. Prescribing should be for the benefit of the patient not the prescriber.

6 Keep up to date about medicines you are prescribing and the related conditions you are treating.

7 Follow CSM guidance on reporting suspected adverse reactions to black triangle drugs and other medicines (see https://www.mhra.gov.uk for links to Yellow Card reporting scheme and downloads of details of reported adverse drug reactions for specific medicines).

8 Ensure continuity of care by keeping the patient's GP (or other preferred medical adviser) informed about prescribing, monitoring and follow-up arrangements and responsibilities.

9 Check that appropriate previous medicines are continued and over-the-counter and herbal medicine use is recorded.

10 Patient Group Directions: the GMC advises these should be limited to situations where there is a 'distinct advantage for patient care ... consistent with appropriate professional relationships and accountability'.

11 Deprescribing should be part of routine patient care. It concerns withdrawing or reducing the dose of medicines, supervised by a healthcare professional. Its aim is to improve outcomes, e.g. by minimising polypharmacy. Deprescribing needs counselling and shared decision-making with patients.

12 Keep up to date with GMC advice on prescribing (GMC guidelines: https://www.gmc-uk.org/ethical-guidance/ethical-guidance-for-doctors/prescribing-and-managing-medicines-and-devices).

13 All sedative medications may impair driving and the ability to operate machinery. Warn patients of this risk.

Common/Useful Drugs

DOI: 10.1201/9781315151816-1

COMMON/USEFUL DRUGS

Notes: Only new or modified drug entries are included here. Some entries have been modified slightly to make them more 'respiratory specific'. Highlighting: Yellow = modification to existing PP text; Green = new drug entry; Grey = important points (for grey box).

ACETAZOLAMIDE/DIAMOX

Carbonic anhydrase inhibitor (sulphonamide-like).
Use: Glaucoma (acute-angle closure, primary open-angle unresponsive to maximal topical Rx, or secondary), ↑ICP. Rarely epilepsy or diuresis. Px for altitude sickness (unlicensed; see page 237).
CI: ↓K+, ↓Na+, ↑Cl– acidosis, sulphonamide allergy, adrenocortical insufficiency, long term in chronic angle-closure glaucoma, **L/R**.
Caution: Acidosis, pulmonary obstruction, renal calculi, elderly R/P/E.
SE: Nausea/GI upset, paraesthesia, drowsiness, mood Δ, headache, Δ LFTs. If prolonged use acidosis (metabolic) and e'lyte Δs. Rarely blood disorders and skin reactions (inc SJS/TENS). For the full list, see manufacturer SPC.
Monitor: FBC and U&E if prolonged use.
Interactions: Many, e.g.: ↑s levels of carbamazepine and phenytoin, may ↓ level of lithium. Can ↑cardiac toxicity (via ↓K+) of disopyramide, flecainide, lidocaine and cardiac glycosides. ↓s fx of methenamine and ↑ fx of quinidine.
Dose: Glaucoma and Epilepsy 250 mg–1 g/day po or iv^SPC (divided doses above 250 mg). Also available as 250 mg MR preparation (as **DIAMOX SR**; max. 2 capsules/day). Diuresis see BNF.

☠ Extravasation at injection site can ⇒ necrosis ☠.

ADRENALINE (im/iv/neb/top)

Sympathomimetic: Powerful stimulation of α (vasoconstriction), β1 (↑HR, ↑contractility) and β2 (vasodilation, bronchodilation, uterine relaxation). Also ↓s immediate mast cell cytokine release.

Use: CPR and anaphylaxis (see algorithms on inside and outside front cover). Rarely: neb for other causes of bronchospasm (e.g. acute severe asthma), partial upper airway obstruction or massive haemoptysis; iv for shock (e.g. 2° to spinal/epidural anaesthesia); top for haemorrhage during bronchoscopy (e.g. airway tumour), adjunct to local anaesthesia.

Caution: Cerebrovascular* and heart disease (esp arrhythmias and HTN), DM, ↑T$_4$, glaucoma (angle closure), labour (esp second stage), phaeo **H/E/R**.

SE: ↑HR, ↑BP, anxiety, sweats, tremor, headache, peripheral vasoconstriction, arrhythmias, pulmonary oedema (at ↑doses), N&V, weakness, dizziness, disturbance, hyperglycaemia, urinary retention (esp if ↑prostate), local reactions. Rarely CVA* (2° to HTN: monitor BP). **NB:** SE still possible with neb or top use.

Interactions: fx ↑d by dopexamine, TCAs, ergotamine and oxytocin. Risk of: (1) ↑↑BP and ↓HR with non-cardioselective β-blockers (can also ⇒↓HR), TCAs, MAOIs and moclobemide. (2) arrhythmias with digoxin, quinidine and volatile liquid anaesthetics (e.g. halothane) and TCAs. Avoid use with tolazine or rasagiline.

Dose: CPR: 1 mg iv = 10 mL of 1 in 10,000 (100 microgram/mL), then flush with > 20 mL saline. If no or delayed iv access, try intraosseous route. Repeat as per ALS algorithm (see front cover). **Anaphylaxis:** 0.5 mg im (or sc) = 0.5 mL of 1 in 1000 (1 mg/mL); repeat after 5 min if no response. If cardiac arrest seems imminent or concerns over im absorption, give 0.5 mg iv slowly = 5 mL of 1 in 10,000 (100 microgram/mL) at 1 mL/min until response – get senior help first if possible as iv route ⇒ ↑risk of arrhythmias.

Neb (e.g. haemoptysis): Use 1 mL of 1:1000 (1 mg/mL) diluted with 4 mL of normal saline.

Top (e.g. during bronchoscopy): Instil 2–10 mL of 1:10,000 (100 micrograms/mL) directly onto the bleeding site through operating channel of bronchoscope.

☠ Don't confuse 1:1000 (im) with 1:10,000 (iv) solutions ☠.

▼ ACLIDINIUM BROMIDE/EKLIRA GENUAIR

Long-acting inh anticholinergic bronchodilator ('LAMA').

Use: Maintenance Rx of COPD (NOT suitable for acute bronchospasm).

Caution: Prostatic hyperplasia, bladder outflow obstruction and angle-closure glaucoma (esp if combined with β₂ agonists; avoid direct exposure of the aerosol and/or powder to the eyes), H/P/B.

SE: Dry mouth (class effect), **paradoxical bronchospasm**, **urinary retention**, **angle-closure glaucoma**, **blurred vision**, constipation, diarrhoea, cough, headache, N&V, GORD, dysphagia, ↑HR, palpitations, AF, pharyngitis/nasopharyngitis/sinusitis, dysphonia. Very rarely dental caries and dry skin.

Dose: 375 μg bd by DPI – equivalent to 322 μg bd of aclidinium (1 puff bd).

 Avoid direct exposure to eyes; risk of angle-closure glaucoma

ALVESCO ICS; see Ciclesonide.

ALTEPLASE

Recombinant tissue-type plasminogen activator (rt-PA, TPA); fibrinolytic.

Use: Acute **MI**, acute massive **PE** (or with haemodynamic compromise, submassive PE). Acute ischaemic CVA w/in 4.5 h of onset (specialist use only).

CI: See page 188 and 248 for use in PE (for use in MI/CVA, see SPC), hypersensitivity to gentamicin, L (avoid if severe)/P/E (acute stroke).

Caution: Any risk of bleeding (inc recent surgery, head injury, stroke [haemorrhagic and embolic] and recent/concurrent use of drugs that ↑ risk of bleeding), external chest compressions, elderly, ↑BP (Rx BP first or concomitantly), recent or concurrent use of drugs that ↑risk of bleeding and conditions in which thrombolysis might give rise to embolic complications (e.g. ↑left atrium ± AF).

L/R/H = Liver, Renal and Heart failure. E = elderly. P = pregnancy. B = breastfeeding.

SE: N&V. **Bleeding** (severe and potentially life-threatening; stop infusion and consider coagulation factors and antifibrinolytic drugs such as tranexamic acid). Reperfusion may → arrhythmias, recurrent ischaemia/angina (MI), pulmonary oedema (with PE) or cerebral oedema (with CVA). Also ↓BP (raise legs and ↓ rate/stop infusion), back pain, fever, uveitis and convulsions. Can cause **allergic reactions** (inc rash, angio-oedema [increased risk with concomitant use of ACEI], flushing and uveitis) and **anaphylaxis**.

Dose: MI: Total dose of 100 mg – regimen depends on time since onset of pain: *0–6 h*: 15 mg iv bolus, then 50 mg ivi over 30 min, then 35 mg ivi over 60 min; *6–12 h*: 10 mg iv bolus, then 50 mg ivi over 60 min, then four further 10 mg ivis, each 10 mg to be given over 30 min. **PE:** 10 mg iv over 1–2 min, then 90 mg ivi over 2 h.

> 🐝 ↓doses if patient < 65 kg; see SPC 🐝. If MI concurrent unfractionated iv heparin needed for > 24 h. Heparin also needed if giving for PE; see SPC.

AMIKACIN

Aminoglycoside: Broad-spectrum 'cidal' antibiotic (see Gentamicin).

Use: Serious Gram-negative infections resistant to gentamicin, pseudomonal infection (e.g. in CF or bronchiectasis) and mycobacterial infection (esp NTM).

CI/Caution/SE/Interactions: See Gentamicin.

Monitor: Check local policy! Amikacin levels: **od dosing regimen** → pre-dose ('trough') concentration should be < 5 mg/L; **multiple daily dose regimen** → 1-h ('peak') serum concentration should be **between 20 and 30 mg/L** and pre-dose ('trough') concentrations < 10 mg/L.

Dose: Consult local policy for dosing! **Od ivi regimen** (NOT for endocarditis, febrile neutropenia or meningitis): initially 15 mg/kg (**ideal Wt for Ht**), then adjust according to levels. **Multiple daily regimen (ivi, slow iv injection or im):** 15 mg/kg/day in two divided dose (can use 22.5 mg/kg/day in three divided doses for severe infection). Doses ≥ 500 mg must be given as ivi. **For both od and**

multiple dosing regimens: max. daily dosage is ≤ 1.5 g for ≤ 10 days (max. cumulative dose = 15 g).

> **NB:** ↓dose if RF and ↑↑ BMI (use ideal or adjusted body weight if obese) and consider ↓dose if elderly. In RF check serum level within range before giving each dose. Adjust dose according to serum levels: call microbiology dept. or pharmacy if unsure. Use eGFR with caution as can over estimate RF, calculate CrCl using Cockcroft and Gault equation.

AMINOPHYLLINE (see THEOPHYLLINE)/NUELIN SA; SLO-PHYLLIN; UNIPHYLLIN CONTINUS; PHYLLOCONTIN CONTINUS

Methylxanthine bronchodilator. *Main Theories of action:* (1) ↑s intracellular cAMP; (2) multiple anti-inflammatory actions; (3) adenosine antagonist; (4) ↓s diaphragm fatigue. NB: additive fx with β₂ agonists (but with ↑risk of Ses, esp ↓K⁺). Aminophylline is a compound mixture of theophylline and ethylenediamine (2:1 ratio) that has ↑H_2O solubility and ↓hypersensitivity relative to theophylline alone.

Use: Maintenance Rx for severe asthma/COPD (po) or acute bronchospasm in asthma/COPD (iv as aminophylline).

CI: Hypersensitivity to any 'xanthine' (e.g. aminophylline/theophylline), acute porphyria.

Caution: Cardiac disease (risk of arrhythmias*), hepatic dysfunction, epilepsy, ↑T₄, ↓T₄, PU, HTN, fever, porphyria, acute febrile illness, **L/P/B/E.**

SE: (Tachy)**arrhythmias***, seizures (esp if given rapidly iv), **GI upset** (esp **nausea**), CNS stimulation (restlessness, insomnia), headache, ↓K⁺.

Monitor: K⁺, serum levels (4–6 h post dose) as narrow therapeutic window (10–20 mg/L = 55–110 micromol/L) but toxic fx can occur even in this range. Also check levels if po dosing.

Interactions: 🕱 NB: has many important interactions (dose adjustment may be needed) and can ⇒arrhythmias (use cardiac monitor if giving iv). 🕱 **metab by P450** (⇒ very variable t₁/₂): **levels**

↑d in HF/LF*/viral infections/elderly, and if taking **fluvoxamine (avoid concomitant use)**/cimetidine/ciprofloxacin/norfloxacin/macrolides (ery-/clari-thromycin)/propranolol/flu vaccines/fluconazole/ketoconazole/OCP/Ca²⁺ channel blockers. **Levels** ↓d in smokers/chronic alcohol abuse, and if taking phenytoin/carbamazepine/phenobarbital/rifampicin/ritonavir/St John's wort. ↑risk of convulsions with quinolones.

Dose: iv: Load* with 5 mg/kg (usually = 250–500 mg) over > 20 min, then 0.5 mg/kg/h ivi, then adjusted to keep plasma levels at 10–20 mg/L (= 55–110 micromol/L). Always follow local policy. If possible, contact pharmacy for dosing advice to consider interactions, obesity and liver/heart function. Po: MR preparations preferred (↓Ses) and doses vary according to brand^BNF. **NB:** ↓**dose** if LF* and dose adjustment may be necessary if smoking started or stopped during chronic treatment.

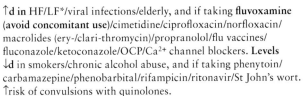

If already taking maintenance po aminophylline/theophylline, omit loading dose* and check levels ASAP to guide dosing. If on a particular brand, ensure this is prescribed as they have different pharmacokinetics ☠.

AMPHOTERICIN/ABELCET; AMBISOME; FUNGIZONE

Polyene antimycotic. Weakens fungal cell membrane by binding to ergosterol. Fungistatic.

Use: Severe, invasive or systemic fungal infections (active against most fungi and yeasts). **NB:** Protein-bound with poor tissue and body fluid penetration.

Caution: **Anaphylaxis** can occur; therefore test dose* is necessary before first infusion. Use in RF if no alternative – contact pharmacist for dose, R/P. Infusion-related reactions can occur and can be severe. Pre-treatment with paracetamol and iv chlorphenamine before each dose and 100 mg iv hydrocortisone before first two doses is recommended.

☠ Fungizone should NOT be used iv as very toxic, only nebulised; for iv use Ambisome or Abelcet ☠.

SE: N&V, abdominal pain, diarrhoea, arrhythmia, Δ BP, chest pain, SOB, headache, ↑T°, Δ e'lyte (inc ↓K+/↓Mg^{2+}), RF, RTA, ↑LFT, haematological (inc ↓Hb, ↓Plt), rash. Less common: anaphylaxis, bronchospasm, neurological (inc convulsions, peripheral neuropathy, tremor, encephalopathy, hearing loss, diplopia), myalgia, arthralgia, TEN and SJS.

Monitor: FBC, U&E (inc K+ and Mg^{2+}), LFT (discontinue if ↑).

Interactions: ↑risk of nephrotoxicity when co-prescribed with tacrolimus, ciclosporin, aminoglycosides or vancomycin. ↑Risk of ↓K+ when given with corticosteroids or diuretics.

Dose: Initial test dose * = 1 mg ivi over 10–30 min. Subsequent doses depend on brand. **Abelcet®:** ivi 5 mg/kg od. **AmBisome®:** ivi 3 mg/kg od. Prolonged Rx (≈ 14 days) is usually indicated.

> ☠ Different preparations are not interchangeable. They vary in PD, PK and dosage. ALWAYS specify brand name in the prescription to be dispensed ☠.

▼ ANORO ELLIPTA

Combination inhaler for COPD. Contains LAMA (umeclidinium) + LABA (vilanterol). See Umeclidinium and Vilanterol.

Dose: Use as DPI. One puff od delivers umeclidinium 55 micrograms and vilanterol 22 micrograms.

APIXABAN/ELIQUIS

DOAC; direct inhibitor of factor Xa. Rapid onset and doesn't require therapeutic monitoring (unlike warfarin).

Use: Px of VTE after THR/TKR; Px of stroke and embolism with non-valvular AF (plus > 1 risk factor, e.g. previous stroke/TIA, symptomatic CCF, DM, HTN or age ≥ 75 years)[2 (BNF)]; Rx of DVT and PE[3 (NICE)]; Px of recurrent DVT and PE[4 (NICE)].

CI: Active or significant risk of bleeding, impaired haemostasis, concomitant use with other anticoagulants, **L** (if severe + coagulopathy)/**P**/**B**.

Caution: Bleeding disorders, active GI ulcer, recent surgery, postoperative epidural catheter (risk of paralysis; monitor neurological signs and wait 20–30 h after apixaban dose before removal and do NOT give next dose until ≥ 5 h after removal), discontinue ≥ 48 h before surgery/procedures with moderate/high bleeding risk and ≥24 h before low-risk surgery/procedures, **R** (avoid if creatinine clearance < 15 mL/min)/**H/E/L**.

SE: **Haemorrhage**, nausea, bruising, ↓Hb, ↓BP, ↓Plt, rash.

Monitor: Hb or signs of bleeding (stop drug if severe).

Interactions: Use of other drugs that increase risk of bleeding inc **NSAIDs**. Concomitant use with strong inhibitors of CYP3A4 and P-gp, e.g. ketoconazole, itraconazole, osaconazole, voriconazole, is not recommended due to ↑ apixaban levels. Strong CYP3A4 and P-gp inducers, e.g. rifampicin, phenytoin, carbamazepine, St John's Wort ↓ apixaban, level by up to 50%. Other interactions possible (consult BNF).

Dose: 2.5 mg bd po, starting 12–24 h after surgery and continuing for 10–14 days if TKR or 32–38 days if THR[1]; 5 mg bd po (2.5 mg bd po if > 80 years + ≤ 60 kg or CrCl < 30 mL/min)[2]; 10 mg bd po for first 7 days, then 5 mg bd po for duration of Rx[3]; 2.5 mg bd po following completion of 3–6 months anticoagulation Rx[4].

AZATHIOPRINE

Antiproliferative immunosuppressant: Inhibits purine-salvage p'ways; prodrug for 6-mercaptopurine.

Use: Prevention of transplant rejection, autoimmune disease (esp as steroid-sparing agent, but also maintenance Rx for SLE/vasculitis, inc pulmonary). Also ILD and sarcoidosis[BTS].

CI: Hypersensitivity (to azathioprine *or mercaptopurine*), severe liver impairment, severe infection, pancreatitis see **P/B**.

Caution: Reduced TPMT activity, **L/R/E**.

SE: **Myelosuppression** (dose-dependent, ⇒ ↑infections, esp HZV), **hepatotoxicity**, **hypersensitivity reactions** (inc interstitial nephritis: *stop drug!*), N&V&D (esp initially), pancreatitis. Rarely cholestasis, alopecia, pneumonitis, risk of neoplasia, hepatic veno-occlusion.

Warn: Immediately report infections or unexpected bruising/bleeding.

Monitor: FBC (initially >wkly for 8 wks, ↓ing to > 3 monthly), LFTs, U&Es.

Interactions: fx ↑ by **allopurinol**, ACE-I, ARBs, trimethoprim (and septrin), DMARDs – ↑risk of myelosuppression, may effect efficacy of intrauterine contraceptive devices (need for additional contraceptive measures), live vaccines (CI), acenocoumarol, febuxostat (concomitant use not recommended), fx ↓ by rifampicin.

Dose: Initially 1–3 mg/kg daily for ≤ 12 wks[SPC/BNF] (preferably po as iv very irritant). NB: ↓ dose in RF, L, and with concomitant use of allopurinol – ¼ of the usual dose of azathioprine given.

> ☠ Before starting Rx, screen for common gene defect that ↓s TPMT enzyme (which metabolises azathioprine) activity: if homozygote for defect avoid thiopurine drugs; if heterozygote, ↓dose (esp if taking aminosalicylate derivatives, e.g. olsalazine, mesalazine or sulfasalazine). Exclude pregnancy before commencing treatment ☠. Counsel patients about teratogenicity and embryotoxicity and need for effective contraception in both women and men before, during treatment and for at least 3 months after stopping treatment. Stop treatment if develop rash, fever or chills, jaundice, bleeding and bruising etc.

AZITHROMYCIN

Macrolide antibiotic: see Erythromycin. Possesses anti-inflammatory ('immunomodulatory') properties.

Use: See Erythromycin (but with ↑activity against Gram-negative and ↓ activity against Gram-positive organisms). Also genital chlamydia and non-severe typhoid. Also used as long-term anti-inflammatory Rx for some patients with asthma, COPD, bronchiectasis and CF (unlicensed indication).

CI: As erythromycin.

Caution/SE/Interactions: As erythromycin, GI sEs, caution in liver disease/L.

Dose: As antibiotic: 500 mg od po *for 3 days only* (continue for 7 days for typhoid); for GU infections 1 g od po *as single dose*. As 'immune modulator' for chronic respiratory disease: 250–500 mg po/od/three times a wk (usually Mon/Wed/Fri); only continue if clear benefit and discontinue if SEs (esp ototoxicity, ↑LFT or ↑QTc); treatment break recommended every 3–6 months; check QTc and LFTs before and after starting treatment.

AZTREONAM
Synthetic β-lactam antibiotic.
Use: Gram-negative infection including *PSEUDOMONAS aeruginosa*, *Haemophilus influenzae* and *Neisseria meningitidis*. Nebulised as azteonam lysine (Cayston®) in CF patients.
CI/Caution: Hypersensitivity to β-lactam antibiotic, **L/R/P**.
SE: Rarely: GI bleeding, colitis (inc C. Diff), ↑LFT, ↓BP, chest pain, SOB, seizures, paraesthesia, confusion, dizziness, asthenia, headache, insomnia, breast tenderness, haematological (inc ↓Plt and ↓NΦ), myalgia, diplopia, tinnitus, halitosis; also reported: N&V&D, abdominal pain, mouth ulcers, taste disturbances, flushing, bronchospasm, rash (inc TEN and EM). **Nebulised drug specific:** Cough, wheezing, dyspnoea, bronchospasm (test dose required), rash, arthralgia, pyrexia.
Monitor: FBC, LFT, U&E.
Interactions: Possible **W+**.
Dose: ivi or iv only (over 3–5 min) – 1 g tds or 2 g bd. Use 2 g ivi tds or qds for severe infections (inc *PSEUDOMONAS* infection if systemic or in CF). **Neb** 75 mg tds.

> 🦵 **RF – Standard initial dose then ↓dose:** eGFR 10–30 mL/ min/1.73 m² ↓half normal dose; eGFR < 10 mL/min/1.73 m² ↓one- quarter normal dose 🦵.

BECLOMETASONE DIPROPIONATE
Inh corticosteroid: ↓s airway oedema and mucous secretions.
Use: Chronic asthma not controlled by short-acting β₂ agonists alone. Also available as nasal preparations (e.g. Beconase®) or po for IBD[BNF].
Caution: TB (inc quiescent).

SE: Oral candidiasis (2° to immunosuppression: ↓d by rinsing mouth with H_2O after use), **hoarse voice**. Rarely glaucoma, hypersensitivity. ↑Doses may ⇒ adrenal suppression, Cushing's, ↓bone density, lower RTI, ↓growth (controversial).

Dose: 200–2000 microgram daily inh (normally start at 200 microgram bd). Use high-dose inhaler if daily requirements are > 800 microgram[SPC/BNF]. ALWAYS specify named product and dose; non-proprietary, **CLENIL MODULITE, QVAR, FOSTAIR** (+ formoterol fumarate 6 microgram), Trimbow (+ formoterol fumarate 6 microgram + glycopyrronium 9 microgram). MDI and DPI devices available. CFC-free pMDI are NOT interchangeable: **QVAR** and **FOSTAIR** contain extra-fine particles and are more potent. Check BNF for delivery devices and doses.

> ☠ Rarely ⇒ paradoxical bronchospasm: can be prevented by switching from aerosol to dry powder forms or by using inh β_2 agonists ☠.

▼ BENRALIZUMAB/FASENRA

Anti-IL-5 monoclonal antibody; reduces production and survival of eosinophils.

Use: Specialist use only. Severe refractory eosinophilic asthma, inadequately controlled despite high-dose ICS/LABA (eosinophil count ≥ 150 cells/µL and ≥ 4 exacerbations requiring systemic corticosteroids in the past 12 months or treatment with continuous oral corticosteroids over the previous 6 months)[NICE].

Caution: Watch for acute and delayed systemic reactions; Screen and Rx pre-existing helminth infections before initiating therapy[BNF]**P/B**. Manufacturer advises Rx pre-existing helminth infections before starting benralizumab. If patient infected during Rx and does not respond to anti-helminth Rx, stop benralizumab until infection resolved.

SE: Back pain; hypersensitivity reactions, eczema; headache; LRTI; nasal congestion; pharyngitis; pyrexia; upper abdominal pain; UTI.

Dose: Use only in specialist centres; for adult, sc into thigh, abdomen or upper arm. First 3 doses 30 mg every 4 wks;

maintenance 30 mg every 8 wks. Remove syringe from refrigerator at least 30 min before administration; avoid injecting into areas that are tender, bruised, erythematous or hardened.

BRAMITOB See Tobramycin.

BRICANYL See Terbutaline.

BUDESONIDE
Inh corticosteroid for asthma[1]; similar to beclometasone. Also available as nasal preparations, or as po and enemas for IBD[2] (see BNF).
Caution: L.
Dose: 200–800 microgram bd inh (DPI only) or 1–2 mg bd neb[1]. ALWAYS specify named product and dose; non-proprietary (e.g. EASYHALER BUDESONIDE), BUDELIN NOVOLIZER, PULMICORT TURBOHALER, SYMBICORT TURBOHALER (+ formoterol fumarate 6 or 12 microgram), DUORESP SPIROMAX (+ formoterol fumarate 4.5 or 9 microgram). Check BNF for delivery devices and doses.

BUDELIN NOVOLIZER
ICS for asthma. See Budesonide.
Dose: Usually: 200–800 microgram inh bd (DPI).

BUPROPION/ZYBAN
Atypical antidepressant; mechanism of action uncertain (can inhibit CNS dopamine, serotonin and NA reuptake).
Use: Aid to smoking cessation in combination with motivational support.
CI: Hypersensitivity to bupropion, history of seizures, CNS tumours, history of bulimia/anorexia, abrupt alcohol/drug withdrawal, severe hepatic cirrhosis, bipolar disorder, concomitant use with MAOIs.

Caution: Avoid or ↓ dose (150 mg po od) in the elderly, liver or renal disease and if predisposed to seizures (inc concomitant use of drugs that lower seizure threshold, alcohol abuse, benzodiazepine or alcohol withdrawal or history of head trauma).
SE: GI upset, dry mouth, agitation, anxiety, depression, headache, rash, pruritis, tremor, sweating, fever, hypertension, insomnia.
Dose: Start 1–2 wks before target stop date: 150 mg od po for 6 days, then 150 mg bd po for 7–9 wks (min. 8 h between doses).

☠ Measure BP before and during treatment (can ↑↑ BP). Warn patient that it may impair motor skills (e.g. driving). ☠

CARBOCISTEINE/MUCODYNE

Mucolytic that ↓sputum viscosity (↓ exacerbation frequency in COPD).
Use: Chronic respiratory conditions with a productive cough (e.g. COPD or bronchiectasis).
CI: Active peptic ulcer disease (can disrupt gastric mucosa).
SE: Rarely GI bleeding, SJS or EM.
Dose: Start as 2.25 g po daily in divided doses (e.g. 750 mg tds po). As condition improves, ↓ to 1.5 g daily in divided doses. Start as 4-wk trial and ONLY continue if beneficial.

Advice patients to stop taking if gastrointestinal bleeding occurs.

CASPOFUNGIN

Echinocandin antifungal; inhibits the synthesis of glucan in fungal cell walls.
Use: Invasive aspergillosis or candidiasis, and the empirical Rx of systemic fungal infection in patients with ↓NΦ.
CI: P/B hypersensitivity to caspofungin.
Caution: L (↓ dose if moderate liver impairment*; avoid if severe impairment).
SE: GI upset (NVD, also constipation, dyspepsia or flatulence), SOB, headache, ↓K+, arthralgia/myalgia, rash, pruritus, sweating, local reactions at injection site. Rarely metabolic (↓pH, ↑Glucose),

Δ LFT, RF, ↓Mg^{2+}, ↓Ca^{2+} or haematological (↓Hb, ↓Plt, ↓ WCC).
Monitor: FBC, U&E, LFT and e'lytes.
Interactions: Levels of caspofungin ↓, e.g. with carbamazepine, dexamethasone, efavirenz, nevirapine, phenytoin/fosphenytoin and rifampicin – use 70 mg dose for whole course; tacrolimus levels reduced – check levels and increase tacrolimus dose.
Dose: 70 mg ivi^{BNF} on first day, then 50 mg ivi od (use 70 mg ivi od if body-weight > 80 kg or if patient taking interacting drug; 35 mg ivi od after first dose if moderate liver impairment*).

CEFTAZIDIME
Parenteral third-generation cephalosporin: Good against
PSEUDOMONAS.
Use: see Cefotaxime (often reserved for ITU setting). First-line β-lactam antibiotic (+ aminoglycoside) for Rx of *PSEUDOMONAS* colonisation or exacerbation in CF or bronchiectasis. Active against *Burkholderia cepacia* (iv or neb).
CI/Caution/SE/Interactions: See Cefaclor and **AAC warning.**
Dose: 1 g tds im/iv/ivi, ↑ing (with care in elderly) to 2 g tds or 3 g bd iv (not im, where max. single dose is 1 g) if life-threatening, e.g. meningitis, immunocompromised. **NB: ↓dose in RF.** For *PSEUDOMONAS* exacerbation or colonisation in CF/bronchiectasis or Burkholderia cepacia: 2 g (3 g if > 55 kg) tds iv (usually 10–14 days).

CHAMPIX See Varenicline.

CICLESONIDE/ALVESCO
Inh corticosteroid for asthma Px, similar to beclometasone but od.
Pro-drug activated in lungs (↓ local and systemic SE).
Caution: L.
Dose: 80–160 microgram od inh (aerosol).

CIPROFLOXACIN
(Fluoro)quinolone antibiotic: Inhibits DNA gyrase; 'cidal' with broad spectrum, but particularly good for Gram-negative infections.

Use: GI infections[1] (esp salmonella, shigella, campylobacter). Also **respiratory infections** (non-pneumococcal pneumonias[2], esp *PSEUDOMONAS*, inc colonisation and non-severe exacerbations in CF/bronchiectasis). Also GU infections (esp UTIs[3], acute uncomplicated cystitis in women[4], gonorrhoea[5]), first-line initial Rx of anthrax.

CI: Hypersensitivity to any quinolone, concomitant use with tizanidine, **P/B**.

Caution: Seizures (inc Hx of, or predisposition to), MG (can worsen), G6PD deficiency, children/adolescents (theoretical risk of arthropathy), patients with history of tendon disease, avoid ↑urine pH or dehydration*, **R**.

SE: GI upset (esp N&D, sometimes AAC), pancreatitis, **neuro-C fx** (esp confusion, **seizures**; also headache, dizziness, hallucinations, sleep and mood Δs), **tendonitis ± rupture** (esp if elderly or taking steroids), chest pain, oedema, **hypersensitivity** (rash, pruritis, fever). Rarely hepatotoxicity, RF/interstitial nephritis, crystalluria*, blood disorders, ↑glucose, skin reactions (inc photosensitivity**, SJS, TEN).

Warn: Avoid UV light**, avoid ingesting Fe- and Zn-containing products (e.g. antacids***). May impair skilled tasks/driving.

Interactions: ↑s levels of theophyllines; NSAIDs ⇒ ↑risk of seizures, ↑s nephrotoxicity of ciclosporin; avoid use with methotrexate as can ↑ methotrexate levels; $FeSO_4$ and antacids*** ⇒ ↓ciprofloxacin absorption (give 2 h before or 4 h after ciprofloxacin), **W+**.

Dose: 250–750 mg bd po, 100–400 mg bd ivi (each dose over 1 h) according to indication[SPC/BNF] (100 mg bd po for 3 days for cystitis); 500 mg po single dose[4]; 100 mg iv single dose[5]. **NB: ↓dose if severe RF.**

> Stop if tendonitis, severe neuro-C fx or hypersensitivity .

CLENIL MODULITE

ICS for asthma; see Beclometasone dipropionate. Available as aerosol inhaler: 50, 100, 200 and 250 microgram.

CODEINE LINCTUS

Oral suspension of codeine phosphate (15 mg/5 mL).

Use: Cough suppressant (opiate).

CI/Caution/SE/Interactions: See Codeine. **NB:** can cause nausea, drowsiness, vomiting, constipation and rashes.

Dose: 15–30 mg tds – qds po, i.e. 5–10 mL (15 mg/5 mL) tds-qds po.

☠ Cough suppression with codeine linctus can cause sputum retention! Use with caution in chronic suppurative lung disease ☠.

COLISTIMETHATE SODIUM (COLISTIN)/COLOMYCIN

Polymyxin antibiotic; active against Gram-negative organisms including *PSEUDOMONAS*, *Acinetobacter* and *Klebsiella*.

Use: Gram-negative infections resistant to other antibacterials[1]. Also by inh (DPI[2] or neb[3]) for chronic pulmonary infection/colonisation with *PSEUDOMONAS* in CF[NICE].

CI: Myasthenia gravis, hypersensitivity to colistimethate sodium.

Caution: Acute porphyria, R/B. With inhalation: bronchospasm* (can pre-treat with SABA, give **after** any other inhaled drugs) and risk of exacerbating haemorrhage during haemoptysis.

SE: iv: Major adverse effects are dose-related **neurotoxicity** (inc apnoea, perioral and peripheral paraesthesia, vertigo, headache, muscle weakness, vasomotor instability, slurred speech, confusion, psychosis, visual disturbances), **nephrotoxicity** and **rash. inh:** sore throat/mouth, taste disturbances, N&V, cough, bronchospasm, dysphonia, thirst and ↑ salivation.

Warn: Discontinue inh if ↑SOB.

Monitor: U&E.

Interactions: ↑ risk of nephrotoxicity and/or ototoxicity when administered with aminoglycosides, capreomycin, vancomycin and amphotericin. ↑effect of suxamethonium and muscle relaxants.

Dose: or ivi[1 BNF] or slow iv[BNF] (only if into a totally implantable venous access device): < 60 kg = 50,000–75,000 units/kg daily in three divided doses; > 60 kg = 1–2 million units tds (max. 6 million units in 24 h). **inh (DPI)**[2]: 1.66 million units bd. **inh (neb)**[3]: 1–2 million units bd.

☠ ALWAYS administer test dose initially, in hospital with pre- and post-spirometry and with access to a bronchodilator* ☠.

COLOMYCIN See Colistimethate sodium (colistin).

COMBIVENT
Compound bronchodilator (salbutamol + ipratropium bromide).
Dose: 2.5 mL (one vial: ipratropium 500 microgram + salbutamol 2.5 mg) tds/qds neb[SPC/BNF].

☠ Protect patient's eyes; acute narrow-angle glaucoma has been reported with neb ipratropium, particularly when given with neb salbutamol (or other β_2 agonists). Use tight-fitting mask ☠.

CO-TRIMOXAZOLE/SEPTRIN
Antibiotic combination preparation: 5:1 mixture of sulfamethoxazole (a sulphonamide) + trimethoprim $\Rightarrow$ synergistic action.
Use: PCP (both Rx[1] and Px[2]); other uses limited due to SEs (also rarely used for toxoplasmosis and nocardiosis). Also used for Burkholderia cepacia, *PSEUDOMONAS* aeruginosa and stenotrophomonas maltophilia, achromobacter, and NTM (unlicensed).
CI: Porphyria, **L/R** (if either severe, otherwise caution).
Caution: Blood disorders, asthma, G6PD deficiency, risk factors for ↓folate, **P/B/E**.
SE: Skin reactions (inc SJS, TEN), **blood disorders** (↓N↓, ↓Pt, ↓Glucose, BM suppression, agranulocytosis) relatively common, esp in elderly. Also N&V&D (inc AAC), nephrotoxicity, hepatotoxicity, hypersensitivity, hyperkalaemia, anorexia, abdo. pain, glossitis, stomatitis, pancreatitis, arthralgia, myalgia, SLE, pulmonary infiltrates, seizures, ataxia, myocarditis.
Interactions: ↑s phenytoin levels. ↑s risk of arrhythmias with amiodarone, may ↑digoxin levels, crystalluria with methenamine,

antifolate fx with pyrimethamine, agranulocytosis with clozapine and toxicity with ciclosporin, azathioprine, mercaptopurine and methotrexate, **W+**.

Dose: PCP Rx[1]: 120 mg/kg/day po/ivi in two to four divided doses for prolonged period (usually 14–21 days). **PCP Px**[2 BNF/SPC]: 960 mg od po (↓ to 480 mg od to improve tolerance; can be given as 960 mg od/bd on alt days (three times/wk). Burkholderia cepacia, stenotrophomonas maltophilia, *PSEUDOMONAS* aeruginosa, achromobacter, NTM RX and Px 960 mg bd po,. Rx ivi 960 mg-1.44 g bd if severe infection **NB: ↓dose if RF.**

> ☠ Stop immediately if rash or blood disorder occurs. Advice patients to report sore throat and fever. Monitor FBC monthly in prolonged courses, in folate deficient pts and elderly ☠.

CREON See Pancreatin.

CYCLOPHOSPHAMIDE

Cytotoxic[1] and immunosuppressant[2]: Alkylating agent (cross-links DNA bases, ↓ing replication).

Use: Cancer[1], autoimmune diseases[2]: esp vasculitis (inc rheumatoid arthritis, ANCA-associated vasculitis and SLE [esp if renal/cerebral involvement]), systemic sclerosis, Wegener's, nephrotic syndrome in children. Occasionally used for 'inflammatory' lung fibrosis associated with connective tissue disease[BTS].

CI: Haemorrhagic cystitis, acute infection, urinary outflow obstruction, **P/B.**

Caution: Acute porphyrias, BM suppression, severe infections, previous or concurrent mediastinal irradiation – risk of cardiotoxicity, **L/R.**

SE: GI upset, **alopecia** (reversible), cystitis, microhaematuria. Others rare but important: hepatotoxicity, nephrotoxicity, blood disorders, malignancy (esp acute myeloid leukaemia), ↓**fertility** (can be permanent), cardiac toxicity, pneumonitis, pulmonary fibrosis (at high doses), **haemorrhagic cystitis** (only if given **iv**: ensure good hydration, give 'mesna' as Px; can occur months after Rx) SPC.

Warn: ↓fertility may be permanent (bank sperm if possible) – need to counsel and obtain consent regarding this before giving. Counsel patients about genotoxicity and mutagenic with need for effective contraception in both women and men before, during and after treatment. Women should not become pregnant until > 12 months after completing treatment, and men should not father a child until > 6 months after completing treatment[SPC].

Monitor: FBC and urine dipstick.

Interactions: Live vaccines (CI), can ↑fx of oral hypoglycaemics. ↑risk of agranulocytosis with clozapine (concurrent use should be avoided) and cardiotoxicity with pentostatin (avoid concomitant use), may ↓ carbamazepine levels (monitor levels).

Dose: Specialist use only. **NB:** ↓dose if LF or RF. Also co-prescribe Mesna (refer to local guidelines), co-trimoxazole (PCP Px) and antiemetics. Ensure good hydration (iv fluids may be required).

> 🏵 Stop immediately if rash or blood disorder occurs. Exclude pregnancy prior to commencing treatment 🏵.

DABIGATRAN (ETEXILATE)/PRADAXA

DOAC (oral anticoagulant); direct thrombin inhibitor. Rapid onset and doesn't require therapeutic monitoring (unlike warfarin).

Use: Px of VTE after THR/TKR[1]; Px of stroke and embolism from non-valvular AF (plus at least one risk factor, e.g. previous stroke/TIA, symptomatic CCF, age ≥ 75 years, DM, or HTN)[BNF,2]; Rx of DVT and PE[NICE,3]; Px of recurrent DVT and PE[NICE,4].

CI: Active or significant risk of bleeding, impaired haemostasis, other anticoagulants[SPC], strong P-gp inhibitors (systemic ketoconazole, ciclosporine, itraconazole and dronedarone)[SPC] **R** – GFR < 30 mL/min, **L** (if severe) **P/B**.

Caution: Bleeding disorders, active GI disease, recent surgery, bacterial endocarditis, anaesthesia with postoperative indwelling epidural catheter (risk of paralysis; give initial dose > 2 h after catheter removal and monitor for neurological signs), weight < 50 kg, age > 75 years (use lower dose), **R** (GFR 30–50 mL/min) **H/E**.

SE: **Haemorrhage**, diarrhoea, nausea.

Monitor: For ↓Hb or signs of bleeding (stop drug if severe).

Interactions: NSAIDs ↑risk of bleeding. Levels ↑P-gp inhibitors (caution with, e.g. amiodarone, clarithromycin, posaconazole, quinidine, verapamil and ticagrelor); levels ↓P-gp inducers (reduced levels dabigatran, caution with rifampicin, St John's Wort, phenytoin and carbamazepine)[SPC].

Dose: 110 mg (75 mg if > 75 years old) 1–4 h after surgery, then 220 mg od (150 mg if > 75 years old) for 9 days after knee replacement or 27–34 days after hip replacement[1]; 150 mg po bd[2]; 150 mg po bd (following ≥ 5 days Rx with parental anticoagulant if DVT/PE)[3,4]. **NB:** ↓dose in RF, elderly or if taking P-gp inhibitors (see interactions).

DEMECLOCYCLINE

Blocks renal tubular effect of ADH. Also licensed for treatment of infections caused by tetracycline-sensitive organisms.

Use: Rx ↓Na+ from inappropriate secretion of ADH (if fluid restriction has not restored Na+ or was not tolerated).

CI: Acute porphyria, tetracycline hypersensitivity, age < 12 years, **P/B**.

Caution: **R** (reduce dose in GFR < 20 mL/min)/**L**

SE: Nausea, vomiting, diarrhoea, photosensitivity (advice patients to wear sunscreen), ↑LFTs, ↑Cr + urea.

Monitor: Renal function, LFTs, signs of overgrowth of organisms, e.g. candida.

Interactions: May need ↑ doses of anticoagulants due to reduced plasma prothrombin activity, absorption impaired by dairy products, food and metallic salts.

Dose: 0.9–1.2 g daily in divided doses (↓ to 600–900 mg daily for maintenance).

DORNASE ALFA/PULMOZYME

Recombinant human deoxyribonuclease (rhDNase); ↓ sputum viscosity by cleaving dead NΦ-derived DNA.

Use: Mucolytic for CF (with FVC > 40% predicted). Specialist use only: 1–3 month trial and assess response (using Sx and spirometry).

Caution: P/B.

SE: Rarely dyspepsia, chest pain, dysphonia, SOB, pharyngitis, laryngitis, pyrexia, conjunctivitis, rhinitis, rash, urticaria.

Dose: Neb (via jet nebulizer, NOT ultrasonic neb): 2500 units (2.5 mg) od.

DUORESP SPIROMAX

Combination inhaler budesonide (ICS) + formoterol (LABA).

Use: Asthma and COPD.

Dose: DPI device budesonide 160/formoterol 4.5 microgram (1–2 puffs bd; max. 4 puffs BD), max. dose only licensed for asthma. Can also be used as MART regimen in asthma (see SPC/BNF). 320/9 microgram (1 puff bd; max. 2 puffs BD), max. dose only licensed for asthma.

▼ DUPILUMAB/DUPIXENT

Recombinant human monoclonal antibody. Inhibits interleukin-4 and interleukin-13 signalling.

Use: Specialist initiation only[BNF/NICE]. Moderate-to-severe atopic eczema[1 BNF], severe asthma with type 2 inflammation (add-on maintenance Rx)[2 BNF], severe asthma with type-2 inflammation (add-on maintenance Rx for patients currently on Rx with oral corticosteroids or patients with co-morbid moderate-to-severe atopic eczema or with co-morbid severe chronic rhinosinusitis with nasal polyps)[3 BNF], severe chronic rhinosinusitis with nasal polyps[4 BNF].

CI: Hypersensitivity to active substance or any excipient. Live and live attenuated vaccines, **B**.

Cautions: Risk of infection from live and live attenuated vaccines and from helminth infection: Rx pre-existing helminth infection before initiating dupilumab Rx; suspend dupilumab Rx if resistant helminth infection develops during dupilumab Rx. live and live attenuated vaccines, **P**.

SE: Eosinophilia, eye inflammation, eye pruritus, headache, oral herpes, anaphylaxis (discontinue Rx immediately), angioedema, arthralgia; eosinophilic pneumonia; vasculitis including eosinophilic granulomatosis with polyangiitis (Churg–Strauss syndrome).

Dose: Use only in specialist centres;[BNF, SPC] initially 600 mg, then 300 mg every 2 wks[1,3] initial dose as two consecutive 300 mg injections at different sites (superscript [1,3]); initially 400 mg, then 200 mg every 2 wks[2], initial dose as two consecutive 200 mg injections at different sites superscript[2]; initially 300 mg, then 300 mg every 2 wks (superscript[4]). Depending on indication, review Rx if no response after 16 wks[1], or yearly superscript[2,3] or after 24 wks[4].

▼ EDOXABAN/LIXIANA

DOAC; direct inhibitor of factor Xa. Rapid onset and doesn't require therapeutic monitoring (unlike warfarin).

Use: Px of stroke and embolism with non-valvular AF (plus > 1 risk factor, e.g. previous stroke/TIA, symptomatic CCF, DM, HTN or age ≥ 75 years)[1 (BNF)]; Rx of DVT and PE[2 (NICE)]; Px of recurrent DVT and PE[3 (NICE)].

CI: Active or significant risk of bleeding, concomitant use with other anticoagulants, impaired haemostasis, AV malformations, oesophageal varices, major intraspinal or intracerebral vascular abnormalities, malignant neoplasms at high risk of bleeding, recent brain or spinal injury, recent brain, spinal or ophthalmic surgery, recent intracranial haemorrhage, uncontrolled severe hypertension and vascular aneurysms, **L** (if severe + coagulopathy)/**P/B**.

Caution: Bleeding disorders, active GI ulcer, recent surgery (discontinue > 24 h before procedure), **R** (reduce dose to 30 mg od po in moderate/severe, avoid if ESRF/dialysis), **H/E/L**.

SE: **Haemorrhage**, nausea, bruising, pruritus, ↓Hb, ↓Plt, rash, abnormal LFTs, headache.

Monitor: Hb or signs of bleeding (stop drug if severe).

Interactions: Use of other drugs that increase risk of bleeding inc **NSAIDs**. Other interactions possible (consult BNF); use lower dose (30 mg od po) with concurrent ciclosporin, dronedarone, erythromycin or ketoconazole.
Dose: 30 mg od po (< 61 kg) or 60 mg od po (≥ 61 kg)[1,2,3].

▼ **EKLIRA GENUAIR** LAMA inhaler for COPD. See Aclidinium bromide.

FLIXOTIDE

ICS. See Fluticasone propionate. **Dose:** (as **ACCUHALER [DPI]** or **EVOHALER** [aerosol]) usually 100–500 microgram inh bd (max. 1 mg bd; dose > 500 microgram bd specialist initiated). Also available as nebules (0.5–2 mg bd neb).

FLUTICASONE PROPIONATE/FLIXOTIDE

Inhaled corticosteroid: See Beclometasone. Also available as nasal preparations (e.g. Flixonase see BNF).
Use: Asthma
Dose: 100–2000 microgram/day inh or 0.5–2 mg bd as nebs. 1 microgram equivalent to 2 microgram of beclometasone or budesonide. Many delivery devices available[BNF]. **ALWAYS** specify named product and dose; available as pMDI (**FLIXOTIDE EVOHALER**), DPI (**FLIXOTIDE ACCUHALER**) or in compound preparations as **AERIVIO SPIROMAX** (DPI; + salmeterol 50 microgram), **AIRFLUSAL FORSPIRO** (DPI; + salmeterol 25–50 microgram), **COMBISAL** (pMDI; + salmeterol 25–50 microgram), **FLUTIFORM** (pMDI; + formoterol 5 microgram), **SERETIDE** (**EVOHALER** pMDI or **ACCUHALER** DPI; + salmeterol 25–50 microgram), **SIRDUPLA** (pMDI; + salmeterol 25–50 microgram). Check BNF for delivery devices and doses.

FLUTICASONE FUROATE

Inhaled corticosteroid: See Beclometasone. Also available as nasal preparations (e.g. Avamys see BNF). Available in combination with vilanterol (Relvar Ellipta) and triple combination with vilanterol and umeclidinium (Trelegy).

FLUTIFORM
Combination inhaler (ICS + LABA): Fluticasone propionate + formoterol. See Fluticasone and Formoterol.
Use: Asthma
Dose: Aerosol inhaler: Fluticasone propionate 50 microgram/ formoterol 5 microgram, 125/5 and 250/10.

FORMOTEROL (= EFORMOTEROL)/FORADIL, OXIS, ATIMOS MODULITE
Long-acting inhaled selective β_2 agonist, 'LABA' (see Salmeterol).
Use: Asthma and COPD. **SE:** as salmeterol and salbutamol plus, **L**.
CI: See Salmeterol/Salbutamol.
Dose: 6–48 microgram daily (mostly bd regime)[SPC/BNF] inh (min./ max. doses vary with preparations[SPC/BNF]). Available as pMDI (**ATIMOS MODULITE**), DPI (noWjan-proprietary, **FORADIL, OXIS TURBOHALER**) or in compound preparations as **FOSTAIR** (pMDI or DPI; formoterol fumarate dihydrate 6 microgram + beclometasone 100 or 200 microgram), **SYMBICORT** (DPI **TURBOHALER**; formoterol fumarate dihydrate 6 microgram + budesonide 100 or 200 microgram; or formoterol fumarate dihydrate 12 microgram + 400 microgram, pMDI formoterol fumarate 6 microgram + Budesonide 200 microgram), **DUORESP SPIROMAX** (DPI **TURBOHALER**; formoterol fumarate dihydrate 4.5 microgram + budesonide 160 microgram or formoterol fumarate dihydrate 9 microgram + budesonide 320 microgram) or FOBUMIX (DPI formoterol fumarate dihydrate 4.5 microgram + budesonide 80 microgram or formoterol fumarate 4.5 microgram + 160 microgram or formoterol fumarate 9 microgram + budesonide 320 microgram) or **TRIMBOW** (pMDI; formoterol fumarate dihydrate 5 microgram + beclometasone 87 microgram + glycopyrronium 9 microgram) or formoterol fumarate 6 micrograms + beclometasone 100 microgram + glycopyrronium 10 microgram).

FORADIL
LABA inhaler. See Formoterol
Use: Asthma and COPD.
Dose: DPI 12 microgram inh bd (max. = 24 microgram bd).

FOSTAIR
Combination inhaler (ICS + LABA; beclometasone dipropionate + formoterol). See Beclometasone dipropionate or Formoterol.
Use: Maintenance Rx in asthma[1] or COPD[2] (lower strength products only, **FEV in 1 second < 50% of predicted**). Also used for MART Rx in asthma (100/6 pMDI only)[3]. **Dose:** as aerosol inhaler or DPI (**NEXTHALER**). Dose varies with preparation[BNF] as beclometasone dipropionate 100 or 200 microgram + formoterol 6 microgram. For 100/6: 1–2 puffs bd[1]; 2 puffs bd[2]; 1 puff inh bd for maintenance + 1 puff inh prn for Sx relief (max. 8 puffs/day; use aerosol inhaler with spacer device)[3]. For 200/6: 2 puffs bd[1].

GANCICLOVIR
Related to aciclovir but ↑activity against CMV.
Use: Local treatment of ocular herpes simplex infection[1]. **Only in immunocompromised patients:** Life- or sight-threatening CMV infection (inc retinitis)[2]; Px of CMV following transplantation[3].
SE: ☠ Very toxic! ☠ **R/P/B.** See aciclovir and consult BNF/local guidelines before prescribing.
Dose: Eye gel 0.15% (1.5 mg per 1 gram[1]) five times/day until healed, then tds for 7 days; Rx ivi 5 mg/kg bd[2] 14–21 days[2], then 6 mg/kg od 5 days/wk or 5 mg/kg od until immunity recovers (maintenance Rx if risk of retinitis relapse; repeat initial induction treatment if retinitis progresses. Px 7–14 days[3]).

> ☠ Ensure adequate hydration and avoid ivi leaks (severe local inflammation/ulceration) ☠.

GLYCOPYRRONIUM/SEEBRI BREEZHALER
LAMA. Similar to ipratropium and tiotropium.

Use: Long-term Rx of COPD.
Caution: See ipratropium + RF, unstable IHD, history of MI, LVF, arrhythmia (excluding chronic stable AF), ↑QT-interval. **Dose:** 1 puff inh od (DPI with 50 microgram capsule); **NB:** NOT for use acutely. Also available in combination with indacaterol (**ULTIBRO BREEZHALER**) or as a triple combination, i.e. **TRIMBOW** (+ beclometasone + formoterol).

HYPERTONIC SODIUM CHLORIDE/MUCOCLEAR®/NEBUSAL®/RESP-EASE®

Used as neb to mobilise LRT secretions. (e.g. CF/bronchiectasis).
SE: Temporary irritation – coughing, hoarseness, bronchoconstriction.
Dose: 4 mL BD, comes in 3%, 6%, 7% (most effective); inh bronchodilator can be used before/after Rx. **ALWAYS check local policy.**

▼ INCRUSE ELLIPTA LAMA inhaler for long-term Rx of COPD. See Umeclidinium.

INDACATEROL/ONBREZ BREEZHALER

LABA similar to salmeterol.
Use: Maintenance Rx of COPD.
SE: See Salmeterol.
Cautions: See Salmeterol, hypersensitivity, epilepsy/seizures, **L**.
Dose: DPI – 150–300 microgram od[SPC/BNF] as DPI **ONBREZ BREEZHALER** (equivalent to indacaterol 150 or 300 microgram/capsule) or in the DPI compound preparations **ULTIBRO BREEZHALER** (equivalent to indacaterol 110 microgram of indacaterol + glycopyrronium 50 microgram/capsule).

IPRATROPIUM/ATROVENT

SAMA bronchodilator and ↓s bronchial secretions.
Use: Chronic[1] and acute[2] bronchospasm (COPD > asthma). Rarely used topically for rhinitis.

SE: Antimuscarinic fx, usually minimal.
Caution: Glaucoma (narrow-angle only; protect patient's eyes from drug, esp if giving nebs: use tight-fitting mask), bladder outflow obstruction (e.g. ↑prostate), **P/B**.
Dose: 20–40 microgram tds/qds inh[1] (max. 80 microgram qds); 250–500 microgram qds neb[2] (↑ing up to 4-hrly if severe). Also available in combination with salbutamol (e.g. **COMBIVENT®**), although better to Rx with single ingredient preparations.

☠ Avoid direct exposure of aerosol to the eyes; risk of angle closure glaucoma ☠.

ITRACONAZOLE/SPORANOX

Triazole antifungal: Needs acidic pH for good po absorption (capsules only; take liquid on empty stomach)*.
Use: Fungal infections (candida, tinea, cryptococcus, aspergillosis, histoplasmosis, onychomycosis, pityriasis versicolor). ABPA in asthma, bronchiectasis or CF.
CI: Hypersensitivity to itraconazole; concomitant use with certain drugs including statins (see BNF for details)
Caution: Risk of HF: Hx of cardiac disease or if on negative inotropic drugs (risk ↑s with dose, length of Rx and age), **L/R/P/B**.
SE: HF, hepatotoxicity**, GI upset, headache, dizziness, peripheral neuropathy (if occurs, stop drug), cholestasis, menstrual Δs, skin reactions (inc angioedema, SJS). With prolonged Rx can ⇒↓K⁺, oedema, hair loss.
Monitor: LFTs** if Rx > 1 month or Hx of (or develop clinical features of) liver disease: stop drug if become abnormal. Levels – trough level after 2 wks rx – 1–2 mg/L. ↑dose if low level.
Interactions: ↓ P450 many; most importantly ↑s risk of myopathy with statins (avoid together) and ↑s risk of HF with negative inotropes (esp Ca² blockers). ↑s fx of ☠ midazolam, quinidine, pimozide ☠, ciclosporin, digoxin, indinavir and siro-/tacrolimus. fx ↓d ++ by rifampicin, phenytoin and antacids*, **W+**.

L/R/H = Liver, Renal and Heart failure. E = elderly. P = pregnancy. B = breastfeeding.

Dose: Dependent on indication[SPC/BNF]. ABPA (unlicensed indication): 200 mg po bd (+ prednisolone). *Take capsules with food (or liquid on empty stomach).* **NB: consider ↓dose in LF.**

IVACAFTOR/KALYDECO (ALSO SEE TEZACAFTOR)

Cystic fibrosis transmembrane conductance regulator (CFTR) protein potentiator that ↑ chloride transport in the abnormal CFTR protein.
Use: Specialist use only. Cystic fibrosis with an R117H CFTR mutation or one of these gating (class III) mutations in the CFTR gene: G551D, G1244E, G1349D, G178R, G551S, S1251N, S1255P, S549N or S549R.
CI: Strong CYP3A inducers, **P/B.**
Cautions: Driving (↑risk of dizziness). Monitor liver function[BNF]. May inhibit CYP2C9: e.g. ↑monitoring on warfarin, glimepiride and glipizide; inhibits P-gp: e.g. ↑monitoring if on digoxin, ciclosporin, everolimus, sirolimus or tacrolimus, **L/R.**
SE/Interactions: Nasopharyngitis, infections (rhinitis, influenza), wheezing, breast abnormalities, diarrhoea, dizziness, ear discomfort, headache, ototoxicity, rash, tympanic membrane hyperaemia, gynaecomastia, ↑blood pressure, hepatotoxicity, ↑blood creatine phosphokinase. ↓dose with concurrent use of CYP3A4 inhibitors. Bitter (Seville) oranges ↑exposure to ivacaftor.
Dose: 150 mg po every 12 h with fat-containing food. If a dose > 6 h late, missed dose should not be taken and next dose taken at the normal time.

☠ See BNF for dose adjustments due to interactions or hepatic or renal impairment ☠.

LEVOFLOXACIN

Quinolone antibiotic. Similar to ciprofloxacin but with ↑activity against *Pneumococci*. Second-line antibiotic for acute infective sinusitis[1], acute exacerbation of COPD[2] and CAP[3], UTI[4] or prostatitis[5].
Dose: 500 mg po/iv od[1,2,4,5] or bd[3] (duration – see BNF/SPC).

▼ LUMACAFTOR WITH IVACAFTOR/ORKAMBI

Lumacaftor improves stability of ΔF508 CFTR resulting in ↑ mature CFTR protein cell surface, while ivacaftor is CFTR protein potentiator → ↑chloride transport.

Use: Specialist use only. Cystic fibrosis patients who are homozygous for ΔF508 mutation.

CI: Strong CYP3A inducers (manufacturer advises ↓ initial dose to 200/125 mg daily for first week), **P/B**.

Cautions: Driving (↑risk of dizziness). Monitor liver function[BNF]. May inhibit CYP2C9: e.g. ↑monitoring on warfarin, glimepiride and glipizide; inhibits P-gp: e.g. ↑monitoring if on digoxin, ciclosporin, everolimus, sirolimus or tacrolimus, **L/R**.

SE/Interactions: Nasopharyngitis, infections (rhinitis, influenza), wheezing, breast abnormalities, diarrhoea, dizziness, ear discomfort, headache, ototoxicity, rash, tympanic membrane hyperaemia, gynaecomastia, ↑blood pressure, hepatotoxicity, ↑blood creatine phosphokinase. ↓dose with concurrent use of CYP3A4 inhibitors. Bitter (Seville) oranges ↑exposure to ivacaftor.

Dose: 400/250 mg po every 12 h with fat-containing food.

> 🐝 See BNF for dose adjustments due to interactions or hepatic or renal impairment 🐝.

MANNITOL

Osmotic diuretic.

Use: Cerebral oedema[1] (and glaucoma[1]). Also used as inh mucolytic for CF ONLY (**BRONCHITOL**)[2]

CI: Predicted FEV1 < 30%, anuria, intracranial bleeding (except during craniotomy), severe cardiac failure, pulmonary oedema, **H**.

Caution: **P/B** – avoid unless essential.

SE: GI upset, fever/chills. Rarely seizures, arrhythmia, oedema, blurred vision, HF. **As inh:** bronchial hyper-responsiveness (test dose first), cough, haemoptysis.

Dose: 0.25–2 g/kg (2.5–20 mL/kg 10% solution) as ivi over 30–60 min, repeated if necessary after 4–8 h (BNF)[1]. **Inh (DPI)** 400 mg bd (first dose 5–15 min after bronchodilator)[2].

MEPOLIZUMAB/NUCALA

Anti-IL-5 monoclonal antibody; reduces production and survival of eosinophils.

Use: Specialist use only. Severe refractory eosinophilic asthma, inadequately controlled despite high-dose ICS and LABA (eosinophils > 0.3 mg/L in last 12 months; four or more asthma excaerbations req. steroids in last 12 months or continuous steroid use of at least 5 mg prednisolone over last 6 months)[NICE].

Caution: Watch for acute and delayed systemic reactions; Screen and Rx pre-existing helminth infections before initiating therapy[BNF] **P/B.** Rx pre-existing helminth infection before initiating mepolizumab. If patient infected with helminth during Rx and does not respond to anti-helminth Rx, stop mepolizumab until infection resolved.

SE: Back pain; hypersensitivity reactions, eczema; headache; LRTI; nasal congestion; pharyngitis; pyrexia; upper abdominal pain; ↑risk of infection (pharyngitis, lower RTI, UTI).

Dose: Use only in specialist centres; 100 mg every 4 wks sc into thigh, abdomen or upper arm.

MOMETASONE FUROATE/ASMANEX

Inhaled corticosteroid for asthma[1]: See Beclometasone. Available as DPI (**ASMANEX TWISTHALER**). Also available as nasal preparations (e.g. **NASONEX**) (see BNF).

Dose: 200–400 microgram/day (bd/on) inh[1] (200 and 400 microgram/dose devices available).

MUCOCLEAR See Hypertonic sodium chloride.

MUCODYNE See Carbocisteine.

NEBUSAL See Hypertonic sodium chloride

NEDOCROMIL SODIUM/TILADE

'Mast cell stabiliser'; unclear mechanism.

Use: Prophylaxis of asthma inc exercise-induced (NOT for acute exacerbations).

SE: Paradoxical bronchospasm (discontinue and use SABA to control symptoms), eosinophilic pneumonia (discontinue), throat irritation, cough, rhinitis and headache.

Dose: 4 mg inh bd-qds; available as aerosol inh (2 mg/mdi).

NINTEDANIB/OFEV

Tyrosine protein kinase inhibitor, antifibrotic.

Use: Idiopathic pulmonary fibrosis if FVC between 50% and 80% predicted[NICE]. Stop Rx if disease worsens by predicted FVC $\geq$ 10% in any 12-month period. Only under specialist supervision.

CI: Allergy to peanuts or soya, P/B.

Caution: Exclude pregnancy before Rx; ensure effective contraception (+ barrier method) during Rx and $\geq$ 3 months after last dose; history of organ perforation or abdominal surgery, history or risk factors for ↑QT, impaired wound healing, ↑bleeding risk, ↑risk of CVD, risk of GI perforation, risk of VTE, L/R (can be severe/fatal – see SPC).

SE: GI upset including abdominal pain, diarrhoea + ↓ appetite, ↓Wt (may need ↓dose if severe); hyperbilirubinaemia, HTN, ↑liver enzymes, epistaxis, rash.

Monitor: LFT before treatment, then monthly intervals for first 3 months, then 3 monthly. If ↑ LFT dose reduction, Rx interruption or discontinuation (see SPC).

Interactions: Levels ↑by ketoconazole; levels ↓ by rifampicin.

Dose: 150 mg bd po; if not tolerated ↓ to 100 mg bd po. **See SPC for ↓dose if SE.**

NICOTINE REPLACEMENT THERAPY/NICORETTE, NICASSIST, NICOTINELL, NIQUITIN

Used for smoking cessation.

Caution: Haemodynamically unstable patients with arrhythmias, recent MI/TIA or stroke, phaeochromocytoma, uncontrolled hyperthyroidism and DM (closely monitor CBG when starting Rx).
Oral preparations: Oesophagitis, gastritis or PUD.
Inhalation cartridges: Asthma/COPD (esp if bronchospastic) and chronic throat disease.
Nasal spray: Can worsen asthma.
Patches: Avoid broken skin +caution with chronic skin disorders. Caution with moderate to severe **L**/severe **R**. **P** (preferable to continued smoking but try smoking cessation without NRT and/or intermittent NRT; avoid patches where possible, but if used ideally remove at night). **B** (present in breast milk but < second-hand smoke, intermittent therapy preferred).
SE: Many. Easy to confuse with effects of nicotine withdrawal. **Mild local reactions** most common, e.g. irritation of throat, mouth or rash. Also paresthesia, ulcerative stomatitis, dry mouth/↑salivation, mouth ulcers, coughing, nasal irritation, epistaxis, sneezing, watery eyes, GI upset may be caused by or exacerbated from swallowing nicotine (GI upset including, dyspepsia, bloating, flatulence, hiccup; oesophagitis or gastritis), palpitations (rarely arrhythmia, e.g. AF), hot flushes, chest pain, abnormal dreams (remove patches before sleep) or arthralgia.
Interactions: Avoid acidic beverages 15 min before use (e.g. coffee or fruit juice) → ↓ absorption of nicotine through buccal mucosa.
Dose: Many different types and methods of administration (see page 229 and BNF).

▼ OLODATEROL/STRIVERDI RESPIMAT
Inhaled bronchodilator: Long-acting β_2 agonist (LABA).
Use: Maintenance bronchodilator for COPD.
SE: Similar to salmeterol + epilepsy/seizures and aneurysm.
Dose: 5 microgram (2 puffs) inh od[SPC/BNF] (as **STRIVERDI RESPIMAT** 2.5 microgram SMI). Also available in combination with LAMA tiotropium (see **SPIOLTO**).

OMALIZUMAB/XOLAIR

Monoclonal antibody that binds to IgE.

Use: Px in poorly controlled allergic asthma[1] (on optimum Rx, have proven IgE-mediated sensitivity to inhaled allergens and require continuous or frequent oral corticosteroids [$\geq$ 4 courses in previous year])[NICE/BNF]. Chronic spontaneous urticaria[2] (severity assessed correctly, not responded to standard tx, reviewed at or before fourth dose, six doses only)[NICE].

CI: P/B.

Caution: Watch for acute and delayed systemic reactions, autoimmune disease, helminth infection (susceptibility), L/R/H/E.

SE: Hypersensitivity/injection site reactions, abdominal pain, headache, $\uparrow$T°, URTI, arthralgia.

Important: Churg–Strauss syndrome (rare).

Dose: Only use in specialist centres; consult SPC[1]. 300 mg sc every 4 wks[2].

ONBREZ BREEZHALER LABA inhaler for use in COPD. See Indacaterol.

OSELTAMIVIR/TAMIFLU

$\downarrow$ replication of influenza A and B viruses by $\downarrow$viral neuraminidase.

Use: Influenza Rx within 48 h of Sx[1]; post-exposure Px[2] ('at risk' individuals, < 48 h after exposure; NOT a substitute for vaccination).

CI: Severe, R (eGFR < 10 mL/min).

Caution: R/P/B.

SE: N&V, abdominal pain, dyspepsia, headache; less commonly arrhythmias, convulsions, $\downarrow$GCS, eczema, rash; rarely hepatitis, GI bleeding, neuroΨ disorders, $\downarrow$Plt, visual disturbances, SJS, TEN.

Dose: 75 mg bd po for 5 days[1] (if eGFR 30–60 mL/min use 30 mg bd; if eGFR 10–30 mL/min use 30 mg od); 75 mg od po for 10 days[2] – Px for $\leq$ 6 wks during an epidemic (if eGFR 30–60 mL/min use 30 mg od; if eGFR 10–30 mL/min use 30 mg/48 h).

OXIS

See Formoterol; LABA for asthma[1] or COPD[2].

Dose: 6–24 microgram inh od or bd (rarely 72 microgram; max. single dose 36 microgram)[1]; 12 microgram inh od or bd[2]. As **TURBOHALER** (6 microgram or 12 microgram as DPI).

PANCREATIN/CREON/NUTRIZYM/PANCREASE/ PANCREX V

Pancreatic enzyme supplement; contains amylase, lipase and protease to assist digestion of starch, fat and protein.

Use: Conditions with ↓/absent pancreatic exocrine function (e.g. CF, chronic pancreatitis, pancreatic cancer or after pancreatectomy or gastrectomy).

Caution: Risk of large bowel strictures (fibrosing colonopathy) with high doses. Urgent review if new/changes in abdominal Sx. Some ↑strength preparations should NOT be used if age ≤ 15 years, e.g. Nutrizym 22, Pancrease HL.

SE: Perioral, buccal and perianal skin irritation (with ↑ doses), N&V, abdominal discomfort (**exclude colonic strictures!**), hyperuricaemia, hyperuricosuria, hypersensitivity (occasionally, if powder handled).

Warn: Ensure adequate hydration (esp higher strength preps). To be taken with food (inactivated by ↓ gastric pH; can prescribe H_2 antagonist or PPI to improve efficacy). NOT to be mixed with hot foods (inactivated by heat). Advise to report any new/Δ in abdominal Sx.

Interactions: Acarbose (antagonises hypoglycaemic effect).

Dose: According to preparation[SPC/BNF] and adjusted in response to patient's nutritional status and the size, no. and consistency of stools. Do NOT forget an extra allowance for snacks. Advice can be sought from experienced dieticians and CF nurse specialist.

☠ Total dose in CF should NOT be > 10,000 units of lipase/kg/day (↑ risk of large bowel strictures) ☠.

PHYLLOCONTIN CONTINUS See Aminophylline.

PIRFENIDONE

Anti-inflammatory and antifibrotic. Mechanism of action not fully understood: known to ↓fibroblast proliferation and ↓fibrogenic mediator production/effects.

Available as 267 mg capsules; 267 mg tablets; 534 mg tablets; 801 mg tablets.

Use: Mild-to-moderate IPF with FVC 50–80%[NICE]; ONLY under specialist supervision; discontinue if disease progression on Rx (↓FVC ≥ 10% in any 12-month period)[NICE].

CI: Concomitant use with fluvoxamine; severe hepatic impairment/ end stage liver disease; GFR < 30 mL/min, **P/B**.

Caution: L/R.

SE: Mainly GI (N&V&D, dyspepsia, GORD, abdominal pain, gastritis, constipation, flatulence); may require ↓dose or Rx interruption. Also ↑LFT, anorexia, ↓Wt, non-cardiac chest pain, hot flush, insomnia, dizziness, headache, somnolence, malaise, distorted taste, URTI, UTI, myalgia, arthralgia, photosensitivity, rash, pruritus, erythema, dry skin.

Warn: Avoid grapefruit juice (↑fx). Avoid direct sunlight, wear high factor sunblock and clothing to minimise sun exposure (photosensitivity rash, can be severe); dizziness/malaise may affect skill performance (e.g. driving); weight loss (take with food to ↓ GI effects); angioedema.

Monitor: LFT before treatment, then monthly intervals for first 6 months, then 3 monthly thereafter; if ↑ LFT dose reduction, Rx interruption or discontinuation (see SPC).

Interactions: ↑ levels by grapefruit juice, fluvoxamine – **AVOID**; levels ↑ by ciprofloxacin (↓ dose; see BNF), to a lesser degree by amiodarone, propafenone, chloramphenicol, fluconazole, fluoxetine, paroxetine. Levels ↓by cigarette smoking, rifampicin.

Dose: 267 mg tds po for first 7 days, then 534 mg tds po for next 7 days, then maintenance Rx 801 mg tds po. **NB:** if Rx interrupted

for ≥ 14 consecutive days, repeat initial 2 wks Rx; interruption <
14 consecutive days → resume at previous dose.

☠ Photosensitivity (see above warning) ☠.

POSACONAZOLE
Triazole antifungal; see Fluconazole and Itraconazole. Better
absorbed than itraconazole. Measure trough levels after few days if
loading dose used – aim for > 1 mg/L.
Use: Second-line Rx for invasive fungal infections or ABPA (with
prednisolone).
Dose: Depends on preparation and indication; consult BNF.
Non-CF patients may need lower doses, e.g. 200 mg daily.

PULMICORT
See Budesonide.
  ICS for asthma. Available as **TURBOHALER** (DPI; 100, 200
and 400 microgram/metered dose)[1], or as **RESPULES** for neb (250
or 500 microgram/mL) suspension. **NOT** suitable for ultrasonic
nebuliser[2].
Dose: 100–800 microgram inh bd[1]; initially 0.25–1 mg neb bd,
then up to 0.5–2 mg neb bd[2].

PULMOZYME See Dornase alfa.

QVAR
ICS for asthma Px; see Beclometasone dipropionate. Aerosol
inhaler (inc breath-activated **AUTOHALER** and **EASI-
BREATHE**; all available as 50, 100 microgram devices). **Dose:**
50–400 microgram inh bd. **NB:** when switching to **QVAR** from
another ICS: if well-controlled asthma, use 100 microgram **QVAR**
in place of 200–250 microgram beclometasone dipropionate or
budesonide = 100 microgram fluticasone propionate; if poorly

controlled asthma, use 100 microgram **QVAR** in place of 100 microgram beclometasone dipropionate, budesonide or fluticasone propionate.

> **NB:** NOT interchangeable with other CFC-free beclometasone dipropionate inhalers; prescribe as brand name ONLY!

RELVAR ELLIPTA

Combination inhaler (ICS + LABA) for asthma or COPD (92/22 microgram strength ONLY); see Fluticasone furoate (NOT propionate) + vilanterol. **NB:** 92 microgram od fluticasone furoate ≈ 250 microgram bd fluticasone propionate. Available as DPI inhaler: fluticasone fuorate 92 microgram + vilanterol 22 microgram and 184/22 microgram devices.
Dose: 1 puff inh od.

▼ RESLIZUMAB/CINQAERO

Recombinant humanised monoclonal antibody. Interferes with interleukin-5 receptor binding: ↓ survival of eosinophils.
Use: Specialist use only. Severe refractory eosinophilic asthma, inadequately controlled despite high-dose ICS/LABA (eosinophils > 0.4 mg/L in last 12 months; ≥ 3 asthma exacerbations requiring steroids in last 12 months)[NICE].
Caution: Hypersensitivity reactions: monitor during and at least 20 min after treatment. Rx pre-existing helminth infection before initiating reslizumab. If patient infected with helminth during Rx and does not respond to anti-helminth Rx, stop reslizumab until infection resolved. Avoid breast feeding during first few days after birth[BNF], **P/B**.
SE: Anaphylaxis, myalgia, secondary malignancy, ↑blood creatine phosphokinase.
Dose: Use only in specialist centres; ivi every 4 wks. See SPC, dose adjusted by body Wt (3 mg/kg). Give intermittently in sodium chloride 0.9% over 20–50 min through an in-line 0.2 micron filter.

▼ RIVAROXABAN/XARELTO

DOAC (oral anticoagulant); direct inhibitor of activated factor X (factor Xa). Rapid onset and doesn't require therapeutic monitoring (unlike warfarin).

Use: Px of VTE for THR/TKR[1], Rx of VTE[2], Px of recurrent VTE[3], Px of stroke and systemic embolism from non-valvular AF (with ≥ 1 of the following risk factors: CCF, HTN, previous stroke/TIA, age ≥ 75 years or DM)[4], prevention of atherothrombosis events after ACS with ↑ cardiac biomarkers (in combination with aspirin ± clopidogrel)[5].

CI: Active or significant risk of major bleeding, recent ICH, malignancy, known vascular aneurysm[BNF] concomitant treatment with other anticoagulants, **L** (if severe or coagulopathy)/**P/B**.

Caution: High risk of bleeding/concomitant use of other drugs that ↑risk of bleeding, severe HTN, prosthetic heart valve (efficacy NOT established), vascular retinopathy, indwelling epidural catheters (follow local policy), bronchiectasis, **L/R/E**.

SE: N&V and haemorrhage; also diarrhoea, constipation, dyspepsia, abdominal pain, ↓BP, dizziness, headache, renal impairment, pain in extremities, pruritus, rash; less commonly: dry mouth, ↓Plt, ↑HR, syncope, angioedema, malaise; rarely: jaundice, oedema.

Warn: Potential risk of bleeding. Advise to take with food.

Interactions: ☠ ↑ risk of haemorrhage when used with other anti-coagulants or anti-platelets ☠. Avoid use with antiretrovirals, azole antifungals (ketoconazole, posaconazole etc.) – ↑ levels/fx ++ (see BNF). Levels/fx ↓by phenytoin, fosphenytoin, phenobarbital, primidone St. John's Wort and rifampicin.

Dose: 10 mg po od, starting 6–10 h after surgery for 2 wks (5 wks if THR)[1]; initially 15 mg po bd for 21 days, then 20 mg po od for duration of Rx (usually 6 months)[2]; 20 mg po od[3,4]; 2.5 mg po bd (usually for 12 months)[5].

▼ ROFLUMILAST/DAXAS

Phosphodiesterase type-4 inhibitor (anti-inflammatory).

Use: Adjunct Rx for severe (FEV$_1$ < 50%) COPD (chronic bronchitis and frequent exacerbations)[NICE].

CI: Moderate/severe hepatic impairment, **P/B**.

Caution: History of depression associated with suicidal ideation/behaviour, pre-existing psychiatric conditions, weight < 60 kg.
SE: Weight decrease, reduced appetite, diarrhoea, nausea, abdo pain (GI s/e usually resolve within few weeks), headache, insomnia, suicidal ideation, depression, panic attack, anxiety.
Monitor: Body weight, change in mood/behaviour, GI tolerability.
Interactions: Cimetidine, fluvoxamine, rifampicin, phenytoin, carbamazepine.
Dose: 250 micrograms od for 28 days then 500 micrograms po od.
NB: Must be started by a respiratory medicine specialist[NICE].

SALBUTAMOL

β_2 agonist, short-acting (SABA): Dilates bronchial smooth muscle (and endometrium). Also inhibits mast-cell mediator release.
Use: Chronic[1] and acute[2] asthma, COPD. Rarely $\uparrow K^+$ (give nebs prn), premature labour (iv).
Caution: Cardiovascular disease (esp arrhythmias*, susceptibility to $\uparrow QTc$, HTN), DM (can $\Rightarrow$ DKA, esp if iv, therefore, monitor CBGs), $\downarrow K$, $\uparrow T_4$, **P/B**.
SE: *Neurological*: Fine tremor, headache, nervousness, behavioural/sleep Δs (esp in children); hyperglycaemia, *CVS*:$\uparrow HR$, palpitations/arrhythmias (esp if iv), myocardial ischaemia, $\downarrow BP$, $\uparrow QTc$*; *other*: $\downarrow K^+$, muscle cramps, lactic acidosis. Rarely hypersensitivity, **paradoxical bronchospasm**. Prolonged Rx $\Rightarrow$ small $\uparrow$ risk of glaucoma.
Monitor: K^+ and glucose (esp if $\uparrow$ or iv doses).
Interactions: iv salbutamol $\Rightarrow\uparrow$risk of $\downarrow\downarrow$ BP with methyldopa, atomoxetine $\uparrow$ risk of cardiovascular SE, caution with digoxin (monitor for signs of AE of digoxin)
Dose: 100–200 microgram (aerosol) or 200–400 microgram (powder) inh prn up to qds[1]; 2.5–5 mg qds 4-hrly neb[2]. If life-threatening, can $\uparrow$nebs up to every 15 min or give as ivi initially 5 microgram/min, then up to 20 microgram/min (according to response and HR). Rarely given po (Step 3 & 4 Asthma Rx): 2–4 mg tds-qds ($\downarrow$dose in elderly).

L/R/H = Liver, Renal and Heart failure. **E** = elderly. **P** = pregnancy. **B** = breastfeeding.

SEEBRI BREEZHALER LAMA inhaler for COPD. See Glycopyrronium.

SEPTRIN See Co-trimoxazole.

SALMETEROL/SEREVENT
Bronchodilator: Long-acting β_2 agonist (LABA).
Use: Add-on for asthma Rx (on top of short-acting β_2 agonist and inh steroids) BTS/SIGN/NICE. **Not for acute Rx!** Also used in COPD.
Caution/CI/SE/Monitor/I: As salbutamol.
Dose: Asthma 50–100 microgram bd inh; **COPD** 50microgram bd. As aerosol inhaler (25 microgram/metered dose) or as DPI **ACCUHALER** (50 microgram/blister). Combination inhalers (+ICS) also available, e.g. SERETIDE, AirFluSal Forspiro, Sirdupla.

SEREVENT LABA inhaler. See Salmeterol.

SLO-PHYLLIN See Theophylline.

SODIUM CROMOGLICATE/INTAL
'Mast cell stabiliser'; unclear mechanism. Similar to nedocromil sodium.
Use: Prophylaxis of asthma inc exercise-induced (NOT for acute exacerbations!).
SE: See Nedocromil sodium.
Dose: 5–10 mg inh qds (can ↑ to eight times daily) as aerosol inh (5 mg/mdi): if exercise-induced asthma can give additional dose before exercise.

▼ SPIOLTO RESPIMAT
Combination inhaler (LABA + LAMA; Tiotropium + olodaterol). See Tiotropium and Olodaterol.

Use: Maintenance Rx in COPD. **Dose:** as SMI (**RESPIMAT**) containing 2.5 micrograms tiotropium + 2.5 micrograms olodaterol; use as 2 puffs od.

SPIRIVA
See Tiotropium; inhaled LAMA.
Dose: 18 microgram inh od by DPI (**HANDIHALER** with 18 microgram capsule) or 5 microgram (2 puffs) inh od by SMI (**RESPIMAT** 2.5 microgram/metered inhalation)

▼ STRIVERDI RESPIMAT LABA inhaler. See Olodaterol.

SYMBICORT
Combination inhaler (ICS + LABA; budesonide + formoterol). See Budesonide or Formoterol.
Use: Maintenance Rx in asthma[1] or COPD[2]. Can also be used for 'MART' Rx in asthma[3].
Caution: DPI (**TURBOHALER**) has different strengths: 100/6, 200/6, 400/12 micrograms).
Dose: 1–2 puffs inh bd, all devices (can be ↑ to max. 4 puffs bd with 100/6 and 200/6 inhalers)[1 BNF]; 400/12 microgram inh bd (2 puffs bd with 200/6, or 1 puff bd with 400/12)[2 BNF]; using 100/6 or 200/6 devices, 2 puffs inh bd for maintenance + 1 puff inh prn for relief of Sx (max. 6 puffs at a time and 8 puffs/day; 12 puffs/day can be used for a limited time)[3 BNF].

TADALAFIL/CIALIS/ADCIRCA
Phosphodiesterase type-5 inhibitor; see Sildenafil.
CI/Use/Caution/SE/Interactions: As sildenafil plus CI in moderate HF and uncontrolled HTN/arrhythmias.
Dose: *For erectile dysfunction*: Initially 10 mg > 30 min before sexual activity, adjusting to response[BNF] (1 dose per 24 h, max. 20 mg per dose, unless RF or LF when max. 10 mg); *for pulmonary*

hypertension: 40 mg po od. Not all brands/generics licensed for all indications.

TAMIFLU See Oseltamivir.

TEZACAFTOR WITH IVACAFTOR/SYMKEVI

Works by improving CFTR (cystic fibrosis transmembrane conductance regulator protein) activity in the lungs. Tezacaftor ↑ presence of the CFTR protein on the cell surface; ivacaftor ↑ function of CFTR, which up arrow chloride transport.

Use:[BNF, SPC] Specialist use only: cystic fibrosis (in combination with ivacaftor) homozygous for F508del mutation or heterozygous for F508del mutation and one of these mutations in the CFTR gene: P67L, R117C, L206W, R352Q, A455E, D579G, 711+3A→G, S945L, S977F, R1070W, D1152H, 2789+5G→A, 3272-26A→G and 3849+10kbC→T.

CI: Hypersensitivity to active substance or any excipient. Strong CYP3A inducers.

Cautions: Monitor liver function[SPC]. P-gp inhibitors, CYP3A4 inhibitors, **L**.

SE/Interactions: Abdominal pain; breast abnormalities; diarrhoea; dizziness; ear discomfort; headache; nausea; ototoxicity; rash; tympanic membrane hyperaemia, gynaecomastia, hepatotoxicity. May inhibit CYP2C9: e.g. ↑monitoring on warfarin, glimepiride and glipizide; inhibits P-gp: e.g. ↑monitoring if on digoxin, ciclosporin, everolimus, sirolimus or tacrolimus. ↓dose with concurrent use of CYP3A4 inhibitors[BNF]. Bitter (Seville) oranges up arrow exposure to ivacaftor and possibly to tezacaftor.

Dose: 100 mg/150 mg tezacaftor/ivacaftor po in the morning with ivacaftor 150 mg po taken separately in the evening.

> ☠ See BNF for dose adjustments due to interactions or hepatic impairment ☠.

▼ TEZACAFTOR WITH IVACAFTOR AND ELEXACAFTOR/KAFTRIO

Improves stability of CFTR to ↑ mature CFTR protein at cell surface (tezacaftor and elexacaftor) plus CFTR potentiator (ivacaftor) → ↑chloride transport.

Use:[BNF, SPC] Specialist use only: cystic fibrosis patients who are homozygous for the F508del mutation or heterozygous for the F508del mutation with any other mutation.

CI: Hypersensitivity to active substance or any excipient. Strong CYP3A inducers.

Cautions: Monitor liver function[SPC]. P-gp inhibitors, CYP3A4 inhibitors (manufacturer advises ↓dose to 2 tablets twice weekly, taken ~ 3–4 days apart and omit evening dose of ivacaftor), **L**.

SE/Interactions: Abdominal pain; breast abnormalities; diarrhoea; dizziness; ear discomfort; headache; nausea; ototoxicity; rash; tympanic membrane hyperaemia, gynaecomastia, hepatotoxicity. May inhibit CYP2C9: e.g. ↑monitoring on warfarin, glimepiride and glipizide; inhibits P-gp: e.g. ↑monitoring if on digoxin, ciclosporin, everolimus, sirolimus or tacrolimus. ↓dose with concurrent use of CYP3A4 inhibitors[BNF]. Bitter (Seville) oranges up arrow exposure to ivacaftor and possibly to tezacaftor.

Dose: 50/75/100 mg tezacaftor/ivacaftor/elexacaftor as two tablets po in the morning with ivacaftor 150 mg po taken separately in the evening. Advice for missed dose: if morning dose > 6 h late, then missed dose should be taken, evening ivacaftor omitted and next morning dose taken at normal time; if the evening ivacaftor dose > 6 h late, then missed dose should not be taken and next morning dose taken at the normal time.

🐝 See BNF for dose adjustments due to interactions or hepatic impairment 🐝.

TIOTROPIUM/SPIRIVA

LAMA for COPD/asthma (Spiriva Respimat only); similar to ipratropium, but only for chronic use.

Caution: Narrow angle glaucoma, prostatic hyperplasia, bladder neck obstruction, RF (eGFR < 50 mL/min/1.73 m^2), arrhythmia[BNF], heart failure[BNF], AMI in previous 6 months.
SE: Dry mouth, urinary retention, glaucoma.
Dose: 18 microgram inh od by DPI (**HANDIHALER**; 18 microgram/capsule) or 5 microgram inh od by SMI (**RESPIMAT**; 2.5 microgram/metered inhalation) or 10 micrograms inh od via Braltus Zonda (10 microgram/capsule). Tiotropium also available in combination with LABA olodaterol (see **SPIOLTO**).

TALC/STERITALC

Sclerosing agent.
Use: Intrapleural administration for chemical pleurodesis following pleural effusion or pneumothorax; see page 215.
SE: Pain (can be severe; co-administration with lignocaine recommended), haemorrhage, ↑T°, ↑HR, SOB, haemoptysis, ARDS (rare).
Dose: Prepare talc slurry (4 g in ≈ 50 mL sodium chloride 0.9%) and administer via chest drain (see page 215).

☠ Monitor for SE and if severe, immediately re-open/unclamp chest drain to allow drainage of talc ☠.

TERBUTALINE/BRICANYL

Inhaled β$_2$ agonist similar to salbutamol. Available as DPI[1] (**TURBOHALER**; 500 microgram/metered dose) or neb[2] 2.5 mg/mL. Can also be given po/sc/im/iv[SPC/BNF].
Dose: DPI 500 microgram od–qds inh[1]; 5–10 mg up to qds neb[2].

TOBI See Tobramycin.

TOBRAMYCIN/BRAMITOB, TOBI

Aminoglycoside: Broad-spectrum 'cidal' antibiotic (see gentamicin). ↑ activity against *PSEUDOMONAS* but ↓activity against certain other Gram-negative bacteria.

Use: See under gentamicin. Primarily used for *PSEUDOMONAS* in CF and bronchiectasis, either iv (with β-lactam or ceftazidime) or inh/neb.

CI/Caution/SE/Interactions: See gentamicin inc ↓dose in RF[BNF]and in pts with ↑↑ BMI (use ideal or adjusted body weight in obese patients) and consider ↓dose if elderly. In RF check serum level within range before giving each dose. Adjust dose according to serum levels: call microbiology dept or pharmacy if unsure. Use eGFR with caution as can over estimate RF, best to calculate CrCl.

SE (specifically for inh): Cough (esp powder), bronchospasm, dysphonia, taste disturbance, pharyngitis/laryngitis, mouth ulcers, ↑saliva secretion, laryngitis, haemoptysis, epistaxis.

Monitor: Tobramycin levels (NOT for inh/neb): pre-dose ('trough') concentration < 2 mg/L; 1-h ('peak') concentration < 10 mg/L.

Dose: By multiple daily dosing regimen (ivi, slow iv injection or im): 3 mg/kg/day in 3 divided doses; can use up to 5 mg/kg/day in 3–4 divided doses if severe infection (but ↓ to 3 mg/kg as soon as clinically indicated). In CF usually 7 mg/kg OD ivi over 30 min. In bronchiectasis or non-CF pts 5 mg/kg OD for *PSEUDOMONAS*. 112 mg (i.e. 4 puffs) bd by DPI inh (**TOBI PODHALER** 28 micrograms/capsule); 300 mg bd by neb (**TOBI, BRAMITOB**).

> **NB:** ↓doses with ivi if RF and with elderly or ↑↑BMI (use ideal or adjusted body weight in obese patients). In RF check serum level within range before giving each dose. Adjust dose according to serum levels: call microbiology dept. or pharmacy if unsure. Use eGFR with caution as it can overestimate RF, calculate CrCl using Cockcroft and Gault equation. Other inhaled drugs should be administered before inhaled tobramycin.

▼ TRELEGY ELLIPTA

Triple combination inhaler (ICS + LAMA + LABA; Fluticasone furoate + umeclidinium + vilanterol). See Fluticasone furoate, Umeclidinium and Vilanterol.

Use: Maintenance Rx in moderate/severe COPD (FEV_1 < 50% predicted).

Dose: As DPI only (ELLIPTA device) containing 92 micrograms/65 micrograms/22 micrograms fluticasone furoate, umeclidinium and vilanterol, respectively, per dose; use as 1 puff od.

TRIMBOW

Triple combination inhaler (ICS + LABA + LAMA; Beclometasone dipropionate + formoterol + glycopyrronium). See Beclometasone dipropionate, Formoterol and Glycopyrronium.
Use: Maintenance Rx in moderate/severe COPD (FEV$_1$ < 50% predicted).
Dose: As aerosol inhaler only (87 micrograms/5 micrograms/9 micrograms of beclometasone dipropionate, formoterol and glycopyrronium, respectively, per dose); use as 2 puffs bd with/without spacer device.

▼ UMECLIDINIUM/INCRUSE ELLIPTA

Long-acting inh muscarinic antagonist used for COPD. Similar to ipratropium and tiotropium, but ONLY for chronic use. Also available in combination with LABA vilanterol (see **ANORO ELLIPTA**) or with ICS fluticasone and LABA vilanterol (see **TRELEGY ELLIPTA**).
Caution/SE: See ipratropium; also cardiac rhythm disturbances.
Dose: Equivalent to 55 micrograms umeclidinium (1 puff) inh od as DPI.

ULTIBRO BREEZHALER

LABA + LAMA combination inhaler for COPD. Hard capsules for inhalation via Breezhaler device. See indacaterol and glycopyrronium.
Dose: 1 puff inh od equivalent to indacaterol 85 micrograms + glycopyrronium 43 micrograms.

UNIPHYLLIN CONTINUS See Theophylline.

▼ VARENICLINE/CHAMPIX

Selective nicotine-receptor partial agonist ($\alpha_4\beta_2$ receptor).

Use: To aid smoking cessation; for smokers who have expressed desire to quit smoking and are part of a programme of behavioural support[NICE].

CI: P/B.

Caution: Previous Ψ history. Patients with a history of seizures, **R**.

SE: GI upset, dry mouth, nasopharyngitis, dyspnoea, cough, taste disturbance, headache, drowsiness, dizziness, sleep disorders, abnormal dreams. Less common include seizures.

Warn/Monitor: Can precipitate (or exacerbate) agitation, depression or suicidal thoughts (esp if previous Ψ history). Can cause hypersensitivity reactions including angioedema; can cause severe skin reactions including SJS, advice patients to seek help if there are symptoms.

Dose: Start 1–2 wks before target stop date: 500 mcg od po for 3 days, then 500 mcg bd po for 4 days, then 1 mg bd po for 11 wks (↓ to 500 mcg bd po if not tolerated; if GFR < 30 mL/min/1.73 m^2 → 500 mcg od po, ↑after 3 days to 1 mg od po). A 12-wk course can be repeated in abstinent individuals to help ↓ risk of relapse[SPC/BNF].

> ☠ Advise patients to discontinue and seek prompt medical advice if they develop agitation, depressed mood or suicidal thoughts; closely monitor patients with history of psychiatric illness ☠.

▼ VILANTEROL/RELVAR ELLIPTA, ANORO ELLIPTA

Long-acting β₂-agonist (LABA): See Salmeterol. AVAILABLE ONLY in combination inhalers with fluticasone furoate (Relvar Ellipta®), umeclidinium bromide (Anoro Ellipta®) or both as a triple combination (**TRELEGY ELLIPTA**).

VORICONAZOLE

Triazole antifungal: See Fluconazole and Itraconazole.

Use: Life-threatening fungal infections or second line for ABPA (+ prednisolone).

SE: As for other triazoles + photosensitivity (must cover up and wear sunscreen) + visual disturbance including poor night vision. Counsel patient that visual disturbance likely transient and not harmful, but if persists consult doctor.

Dose: Depends on preparation and indication; consult BNF. Measure trough levels after 7 days – 1.3–4.7 mg/L.

XOLAIR See Omalizumab.

ZYBAN See Bupropion.

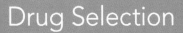

Drug Selection

DOI: 10.1201/9781315151816-2

ANTIMICROBIALS

Important points:

- The following are only guides to a rational start to Rx. Local organisms, sensitivities and prescribing preferences vary widely, with most UK hospitals now providing antibiotic and antimicrobial protocols: if unsure, consult your microbiology department/pharmacy.
  - Empirical ('best guess') Rx is given unless stated otherwise.
  - To decide if 'severe' Rx is necessary, consider each individual's comorbidity, assess clinical features, apply any available severity scores and consider whether you have time to give simple Rx first, before adding/changing if the patient fails to improve.
  - Many antifungals/antibacterials ↓/↑ P450; therefore, always consider potential for drug interactions.
- Always get as many appropriate cultures as possible *before* starting Rx (e.g. sputum or blood); if unfamiliar with patient, checking for recent culture results could help aid choice of agent.
- When prescribing: always specify the indication and intended duration, narrow the spectrum if specific organisms are identified or clinical condition allows, review the need for IV Rx daily and consider stopping Rx or de-escalating to PO as soon as possible.
- ALWAYS consider whether an infectious disease or causative organism are notifiable under the Health Protection (Notification) Regulations 2010 (page 284); medical practitioners have a statutory duty to notify the 'proper officer' at the local council or local health protection team.

It is essential to ask each patient in person about allergies before prescribing. Do not rely on notes or drug charts, which are often incomplete or inaccurate. Remember: If you prescribe it, you are liable! If the patient is unconscious, check the notes thoroughly (or contact relatives/GP if time). Do not let an incident (or near-incident) be the way you learn this!

PNEUMONIA
Please see Respiratory Emergencies (page 256).

UPPER RESPIRATORY TRACT INFECTIONS
Acute pharyngitis and tonsillitis
Mainly viral with two bacterial infections caused by group A
streptococci, *Streptococcus pneumoniae* or *Haemophilus influenzae*.
Distinguish from infectious mononucleosis (Epstein–Barr Virus).
Treatment: Usually supportive. Antibiotics only required if
bacterial infection confirmed, or if three of the following four
clues present: purulent tonsils, fever, lack of cough or cervical
lymphadenopathy. Use penicillin v (phenoxymethylpenicillin)
500 mg qds po. ☠ Hypersensitivity reactions can occur with
β-lactams if infectious mononucleosis ☠.

Acute epiglottitis
Infection localised to epiglottis and surrounding structures.
Resulting oedema can be life-threatening. ☠ Beware stridor! ☠.
Causative microorganisms are *streptococci*, *S. pneumoniae* or
H. influenzae.
Treatment: Cefotaxime 1 g tds iv ± metronidazole 500 mg tds iv
(or TAZOCIN [piperacillin + tazobactam] 4.5 g tds iv).

Acute bronchitis, tracheitis and tracheobronchitis
Inflammation of the trachea and/or bronchial tree. Typically
follows a viral infection. Two bacterial infections are common,
particularly with *S. pneumoniae* or *H. influenzae*.
Treatment: Supportive. Antibiotics usually not indicated, unless
two infections suspected.

EMPYEMA
Pus in the pleural cavity. ☠ Always consider in patients with
CAP who are failing to improve ☠. Pleural infection can
occur, however, in the absence of a preceding pneumonic illness
('1 empyema'). Empyema and parapneumonic effusion require
urgent pleural aspiration → if fluid is purulent, turbid, pH < 7.2 or
cultures organisms, it requires urgent drainage.

Treatment: As for CAP or HAP (page 256). Consider + metronidazole 500 mg tds iv for anaerobic cover. Rationalise and narrow spectrum once culture results (**NB:** significant proportion may be culture negative). Prolonged antibiotic Rx is recommended (3–4 wks). Change IV → PO antibiotics only once afebrile and clinical improvement. Chest tube drainage is urgently required ± surgery (VATS or decortication) and nutritional support. Intrapleural streptokinase (fibrinolytic; unlicensed indication) is occasionally advisable for very purulent and loculated empyema (instil 250,000 IU in 30–50 mL normal saline bd), but only after specialist advice!

Lung abscess

A localised area of pulmonary suppuration ± cavity formation. May be single or multiple, acute or chronic (> 6 wks), 1 (1 lung infection) or 2 (result of another condition or colonisation of a pre-existing cavity). Can be life-threatening and result in complications such as haemoptysis, empyema or bronchopleural fistula.

Treatment: Seek microbiology advice! Infection can be mixed, so broad-spectrum often required. Start Co-amoxiclav 1.2 g tds iv (or clindamycin with cephalosporin). Consider + metronidazole 500 mg tds iv to cover anaerobes. Common practice is Rx for 1–2 wks iv with a further 4 wks po. Additional Rx, such as percutaneous drainage or surgery may also be required.

OTHER RARE BACTERIAL LUNG INFECTIONS
Nocardiosis

Consider *Nocardia* when pulmonary infection presents with soft tissue abscess ± CNS infection (meningitis ± abscess).

Treatment: Always consult infectious disease specialist! Long-term (6–12 months) Rx with sulphonamide, e.g. co-trimoxazole is recommended.

Actinomycosis

Consider when pulmonary symptoms accompany extra-pulmonary infection (particularly head and neck, e.g. mandible) in an immunocompromised patient.

Treatment: Always consult infectious disease specialist! Long-term (6–12 months) Rx with a penicillin.

Melioidosis
Consider infection with *Burkholderia pseudomallei* in returning travellers from Asia (esp Thailand) or Australia with CAP or a subacute (TB-like) illness.

Treatment: Always consult infectious disease specialist! Use ceftazidime 2 g tds iv for first 14 d, then co-trimoxazole po for at least 12 wks.

Leptospirosis ('Weil's disease')
Transmitted from water or soil contaminated with urine of infected animals (e.g. rats) coming in contact with broken skin or mucosal surfaces. Ranges from mild symptoms to pneumonia and diffuse pulmonary haemorrhage.

Treatment: Always consult infectious disease specialist! Antibiotic of choice is typically a penicillin (e.g. benzyl-penicillin).

ASPERGILLUS
Aspergillus is a ubiquitous fungus that is ↑ isolated with ↑ indoor humidity. Inhalation of spores can result in a variety of different conditions (see Box).

Allergic bronchopulmonary aspergillosis (ABPA)
ABPA is a hypersensitivity response to aspergillus in airways → inflammation and damage of bronchial walls ± bronchiectasis. Seen most commonly in asthmatics and CF. Main diagnostic criteria are: asthma, proximal bronchiectasis, +ve skin prick/IgE to *A. fumigatus* and IgG to *A. fumigatus*.

A. fumigatus – Pulmonary conditions

1 **Atopy** – IgE-mediated allergy to aspergillus
2 **Allergic Bronchopulmonary Aspergillosis (ABPA)**
3 **Aspergilloma**
4 **Chronic Necrotising Aspergillosis**
5 **Invasive Aspergillosis**

Treatment: Optimise asthma treatment (inc ICS). Long courses of prednisolone + itraconazole 200 mg po bd (works as a steroid sparing agent). Alternatives: voriconazole, Posaconazole or Isavuconazole (last line) (seek advice before commencing). ALWAYS check LFTs before starting and during treatment. Check antifungal levels (refer to local policy).

Aspergilloma (Mycetoma)

A ball of fungal hyphae in a pre-existing lung cavity (typical from TB). Often asymptomatic but can cause chronic or massive haemoptysis.
Treatment: May not be required. If symptomatic: itraconazole 200 mg bd po may ↓ size of aspergilloma. ALWAYS check LFTs before starting and during treatment. Check antifungal levels (refer to local policy). Manage haemoptysis (page 244); may need to consider arterial embolization ± surgery.

Chronic necrotising aspergillosis

Also known as semi-invasive aspergillosis. An indolent pneumonia that is unresponsive to antibiotics. Ranges from patchy consolidation to cavitating pneumonia. Suspect in patients with mild immunosuppression (e.g. DM, steroids, chronic lung disease).
Treatment: Use itraconazole 200 mg po bd. Unlike ABPA however, steroids NOT recommended (risk of further immunosuppression). Alternatives: Voriconazole, Posaconazole or Isavuconazole (last line) (seek advice before commencing). ALWAYS Check LFTs before starting and during treatment. Check antifungal levels (refer to local policy).

Invasive aspergillosis

Aspergillus hyphae invade tissue. Usually after severe immunosuppression (e.g. chemotherapy with ↓Nɸ). Consider when ↑T° and pulmonary infiltrates failing to respond to broad-spectrum antibiotics. Can disseminate to other organs.
Treatment: ↑ Mortality; start antifungal early and urgently consult microbiology. Options include: Liposomal Amphotericin B (AmBisome) 1 mg/kg/d on day 1 then ↑ to 3 mg/kg/d if tolerated

(**ALWAYS** use test dose first: 1 mg over 10 min then observe for
30 min). Monitor LFTs, RF, U&Es. Consider pre-medication
30 min before each dose with hydrocortisone 100 mg iv (if not on
corticosteroids; first two doses), paracetamol and chlorphenamine
10 mg iv.

PNEUMOCYSTITIS PNEUMONIA (PCP)

Pneumonia resulting from infection with the fungus *Pneumocystis
jiroveci* (previously *Pneumocystis carinii*). Typically seen in HIV
infection (CD4 $< 200 \times 10^6$/L). Hypoxia and $\downarrow O_2$ sats on exercise
suggests PCP in HIV positive patients. Diagnosis is by identification
of *Pneumocystis jiroveci* in induced sputum or bronchoalveolar
lavage.
Treatment: High-dose co-trimoxazole 120 mg/kg/24 h po/iv
(in four divided doses). Continue for 2–3 wks. Also use high-dose
prednisolone 40 mg bd po, if respiratory failure, for 5–7 d then
taper. Start HAART.

VIRAL PNEUMONIA

Viral URTI is common, but viral pneumonia is unusual and typically
only seen in the elderly, children and immunocompromised.
Influenza is the most common virus. Others include cytomegalovirus
(CMV), varicella, respiratory syncytial virus (RSV) and measles.
Bacterial secondary infection can also occur (Rx as per CAP; page 256).
Pandemics of some influenza strains (H1N1 ['Swine Flu'] and
H5N1/H7N9 ['Avian Flu']) and coronavirus ('SARS') have occurred
globally in recent years. **NB:** clinical and radiological features are
often non-specific. ☠ Viral pneumonia can be life threatening! ☠

Influenza

Seasonal influenza well recognised in UK (winter months).
Incubation is 1–4 d; adults are contagious for 1 wk. 'Flu' with
URTI Sx are most common. LRT complications inc bronchitis
and 1 viral pneumonia (2 bacterial infection is more common).
Diagnosis should be suspected with bilateral mid-zone interstitial
infiltrates on CXR. Consider pandemic flu with appropriate Hx.

Treatment: Mainly supportive. Always check local policies and guidance on antiviral Rx for seasonal and pandemic influenza. Consider oseltamivir (TAMIFLU) 75 mg bd po for 5 d in 'at risk' patients, < 48 h after symptom onset. It ↓s length of symptoms.

Influenzae – 'At Risk' Individuals

1 Age > 65 years
2 Pregnant women
3 Chronic respiratory disease (inc. asthma and COPD)
4 Chronic heart disease
5 Chronic renal disease
6 Chronic liver disease
7 Chronic neurological disease
8 Immunosuppression
9 Diabetes mellitus

Cytomegalovirus (CMV) pneumonia

Commonest viral pathogen in immunocompromised, esp following organ transplantation. Infection can also result from reactivation of latent CMV. ↑ mortality.

Treatment: Ganciclovir 5 mg/kg bd iv for 14–21 d. Beware ↓Nϕ and ↓Hb (regularly check FBC). If viral resistance; foscarnet 60 mg/kg iv tds. Consider hyperimmune globulin or valganciclovir 900 mg BD po with severe or relapsed CMV.

Varicella pneumonia

Rarely occurs during chickenpox or shingles. Pregnant and immunocompromised at ↑ risk. Often resolves spontaneously but can progress to respiratory failure and death!

Treatment: Isolation. Early Rx with aciclovir 10 mg/kg tds iv for 7 d. NOT licensed in pregnancy but benefit > risk, so should be considered. Varicella-zoster Ig for immunocompromised and pregnant.

Respiratory syncytial virus (RSV)

Very common cause of pneumonia and bronchiolitis in children. Less common in adults (usually the chronically unwell).

Treatment: Supportive. May be role for neb ribavirin (VIRAZOLE); check local policies.

Measles
Very rare in adults.
Treatment: Supportive.

Coronavirus
Pulmonary infection with SARS coronavirus (SARS-CoV) → severe acute respiratory syndrome (SARS). SARS-CoV was the cause of a large pandemic between 2002 and 2003, but is no longer a threat to public health. SARS-CoV-2 has been the cause of a global pandemic since 2019 (COVID-19). Other CoV, e.g. Middle East respiratory syndrome coronavirus (MERS-CoV) could result in future global pandemics.
Treatment: Supportive. Benefit from anti-viral treatment is unknown. On-going studies to look at potential treatments for COVID-19, including the role of systemic corticosteroids (increasingly used as either dexamethasone or prednisolone to Rx pneumonitis/organising pneumonia).

ASTHMA

Heterogeneous respiratory disorder characterised by airway inflammation and bronchial hyper-reactivity. Variable (reversible) airflow obstruction is seen (**NB:** can become irreversible over time, i.e. 'Asthma with Fixed Airflow Obstruction'). A subset are eosinophilic and/or atopic (react to specific aeroallergens). The diagnosis is clinical but should be supported by objective measures: PEFR diary with diurnal variation, bronchodilator reversibility testing, peripheral eosinophilia, raised total IgE or IgE/skin prick testing specific to various aeroallergens (e.g. house dust mite). More specialised tests, such as metacholine challenges or bronchial provocation may be required when diagnosis uncertain. Exhaled nitric oxide (FeNO) provides a quantitative assessment of airways inflammation and can act as a biomarker to assess the response to treatments such as ICS and/or monoclonal antibodies (e.g. mepolizumab): < 25 ppb (low), 25–50 ppb (intermediate), > 50 ppb (high); **NB:** a raised FeNO (> 25 ppb) increases the probability of asthma, but a normal FeNO (< 25 ppb) does not exclude asthma and changes of 10 ppb (or 20% are considered significant).

NON-PHARMACOLOGICAL TREATMENT

Very important to consider and advise: *allergen avoidance* (esp house dust mite), *smoking cessation* and *weight reduction* (weight loss correlates with better asthma control).

PHARMACOLOGICAL TREATMENT

Aim of Rx is to achieve disease control, i.e. no Sx, no need for rescue Rx and normal spirometry. A stepwise approach is used, using the latest guidance[BTS/NICE/SIGN or GINA]. Start at the step most appropriate to initial severity of asthma and sequentially move up Rx steps until control is achieved. Figure 2.1 is an example of a stepwise approach. **Important: before initiating a new Rx, always check adherence, inhaler technique and allergen avoidance FIRST. ALWAYS remember to 'step down' Rx when disease control is achieved.**

Inh short-acting β_2 agonist PRN (SABA; 'reliever') is generally prescribed for all asthmatics; most commonly by pressurised metered-dose inhaler (pMDI) (± spacer to improve delivery), using salbutamol 100–200 micrograms (1–2 puffs) PRN, or terbutaline 500 micrograms (1 puff) PRN. May be appropriate to manage patients without SABA and using MART therapy (discussed hereunder)[GINA].

Regular preventer therapy: Many patients (ALWAYS those with evidence of airway inflammation, i.e. raised FeNO) will require ICS (**'preventer'**). Other indications for starting ICS include: (1) using SABA ≥ 3 times/wk; (2) Sx ≥ 3 times/wk; (3) waking ≥ 1 time/wk; (4) otherwise poor asthma control (e.g. as adjudged by the asthma control questionnaire); (5) asthma attack in last 2 yrs. Options: **Beclometasone dipropionate (BDP), budesonide, ciclesonide, fluticasone propionate,** or **mometasone furoate.** For

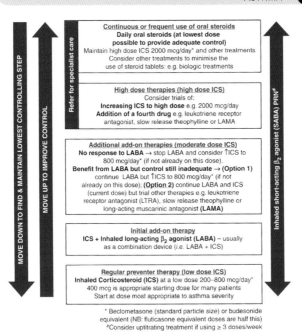

Figure 2.1 BTS & SIGN guidelines on the management of asthma 2016 (Adapted from BTS website).

most patients start 400 micrograms/d (BDP equivalent) and titrate until asthma controls. Almost all (except ciclesonide) are prescribed bd. Beclometasone ≈ budesonide in clinical practice (assume 1:1 ratio). Ciclesonide, fluticasone and mometasone provide equal clinical activity at half the BDP dosage. Higher doses may be required for smokers or ex-smokers. Doses < 800 micrograms BDP only associated with local SE (e.g. candidiasis or dysphonia). ↓ Bone mineral density and adrenal suppression should be considered with

↑ doses. Ciclesonide (ALVESCO) is a lung-activated pro-drug and may result in ↓ local and systemic side effects. It is commonly prescribed alongside an ICS/LABA combination to achieve higher doses of ICS without side effects from the increased LABA (e.g. Fostair 200/6 mcg inh 2 puffs bd + ciclesonide 160 mcg inh 1 puff od). QVAR (BDP) has a smaller particle size and may benefit some asthmatics. **VITAL:** ICS-containing inhalers should always be prescribed by brand to ensure the patient receives the correct device.

Add-on therapies: Add inh *long-acting β₂ agonist (LABA)* without discontinuing ICS. Consider addition of LABA with ICS doses > 400 micrograms BDP and always start if > 800 micrograms BDP. Combination inhalers (ICS-LABA) guarantee LABA is taken with ICS and may improve inhaler adherence, e.g. FOSTAIR or SYMBICORT. ICS-LABA are the preferred initial devices for this step in asthma treatment. ☠ Ensure clinically effective dosage of ICS is *not* ↓ inadvertently when converting ICS to ICS-LABA device ☠. *Maintenance & Reliever Therapy (MART)* can also be considered: adults who are poorly controlled and using ICS-LABA combination device as preventer (e.g. SYMBICORT or FOSTAIR) can also use this combination device as their reliever (ensuring daily ICS dosage not exceeded). If no response to LABA → discontinue and ↑ICS to 800 micrograms. If some response to LABA but asthma control still inadequate → continue LABA and ↑ICS to 800 micrograms *or* continue with the current ICS dose (+LABA) and try adding in a second-line therapy: leukotriene receptor antagonist montelukast 10 mg on po (SINGULAIR), slow-release theophylline (SLO-PHYLLIN 250–500 mg bd po, UNIPHLLIN CONTINUS 200–400 mg bd po) or a long-acting muscarinic antagonist (LAMA), e.g. tiotropium SMI 5 micrograms (2 puffs) inh od (SPIRIVA RESPIMAT). Oral slow-release β₂ agonists can be trialled but are rarely used.

High-dose therapies: If control remains inadequate despite ICS (800 micrograms BDP) + LABA and/or additional add-on therapies, consider a trial of: (1) ↑ dose ICS to 2000 micrograms BDP; (2) Addition of a fourth drug: leukotriene receptor antagonist

Table 2.1 Inhaled corticosteroid quick reference guide

Beclometasone dipropionate (BDP)

Aerosol

Non-proprietary	400 micrograms BDP	See individual preparations
CLENIL MODULATE	400 micrograms BDP	50, 100, 200 & 250 micrograms devices
QVAR	200 micrograms BDP	50 & 100 micrograms AUTOHALER or EASI-BREATH breath-actuated devices
FOSTAIR (ICS/LABA; + formoterol)	200 micrograms BDP	100/6 & 200/6 micrograms devices

Dry powder

ASMABEC CLICKHALER	400 micrograms BDP	100 & 250 micrograms devices
FOSTAIR NEXTHALER (ICS/LABA; + formoterol)	200 micrograms BDP	100/6 & 200/6 micrograms devices

Budesonide

Dry powder

Non-proprietary (e.g. EASYHALER)	400 micrograms BDP	100, 200 & 400 micrograms devices
BUDELIN NOVOLIZER	400 micrograms BDP	200 micrograms devices
PULMICORT TURBOHALER	400 micrograms BDP	100, 200 & 400 micrograms devices
SYMBICORT TURBOHALER (ICS/LABA; + formoterol)	400 micrograms BDP	100/6, 200/6 & 400/12 micrograms devices
DUORESP SPIROMAX (ICS/LABA; + formoterol)	400 micrograms BDP	160/4.5 & 320/9 micrograms devices

Ciclesonide

Aerosol

ALVESCO	200–300 micrograms BDP	80 & 160 micrograms devices

(Continued)

Table 2.1 Inhaled corticosteroid quick reference guide (*Continued*)

Fluticasone propionate

Aerosol

FLIXOTIDE EVOHALER	200 micrograms BDP	50, 125 & 250 micrograms devices
FLUTIFORM (ICS/LABA; + formoterol)	200 micrograms BDP	50/5, 125/5 & 250/10 micrograms devices
SERETIDE EVOHALER (compound; + salmeterol)	200 micrograms BDP	50, 125 & 250 micrograms devices

Dry powder

FLIXOTIDE ACCUHALER	200 micrograms BDP	50, 100, 250 & 500 micrograms devices
SERETIDE ACCUHALER (ICS/LABA; + salmeterol)	200 micrograms BDP	100, 250 & 500 micrograms devices

Fluticasone furoate

Dry powder

RELVAR ELLIPTA (ICS/LABA; + vilanterol)	92 micrograms od approximately equivalent to 250 micrograms bd fluticasone propionate	92/22 & 184/22 micrograms devices

Mometasone furoate

Dry powder

ASMANEX TWISTHALER	200 micrograms BDP	200 & 400 micrograms devices

(discussed ealier), slow-release theophylline (discussed ealier), LAMA (discussed ealier) or slow-release oral β_2 agonist. Practically, higher doses of ICS can be achieved by adding in a pure ICS device alongside the patient's regular ICS/LABA combination device (avoids any side effects from LABA over-use). ALWAYS use a spacer when prescribing high doses of ICS via pMDI.

Continuous or frequent use of steroids: A small number of patients require either the daily use or regular prescription of oral steroids to maintain asthma control. Use lowest possible dose of prednisolone. ☠ **Monitor:** BP, BM, lipids & bone mineral density. **Co-prescribe:** bisphosphonate (alendronate 10 mg po wkly) ☠. Also check vitamin D level and supplement if necessary.

'Difficult-to-treat' and severe asthma: Some patients have persistent symptoms and/or exacerbate despite high-dose ICS and/or regular or continuous use oral steroids. Essential to systematically re-assess the diagnosis, Rx adherence and psychosocial factors. Also assess for co-existing disease (e.g. ABPA, bronchiectasis, EDAC, vocal cord dysfunction). Such patients should be assessed in a specialist centre. Those with evidence of persistent airway inflammation despite high-dose ICS are referred to as **severe asthma** and should be considered for other Rx, as discussed here (e.g. anti-Il-5 mAbs). Those without evidence of persistent Th2 inflammation are referred to as '**difficult-to-treat**' asthma and alternative explanations for their symptoms should be sought (as discussed earlier).

OTHER TREATMENTS

- *IM steroids* may be helpful if poor compliance with inhaled therapy or oral prednisolone, e.g. triamcinolone 120 mg.
- *Anti-IgE monoclonal antibody* (Omalizumab, XOLAIR) for those with severe asthma who are atopic (aeroallergen sensitised) and are symptomatic/regularly exacerbate despite high-dose ICS. Given as SC injection according to body weight and IgE concentration every 2–4 wks. Use ONLY in specialised centre.
- *Anti-interleukin-5 monoclonal antibodies* are used for patients with evidence of poorly controlled severe eosinophilic asthma. They include Mepolizumab (NUCALA), Reslizumab (CINQAERO) and Benralizumab (FASENRA). Mepolizumab (100 mg sc every 4 wks) is approved for use in asthmatics who have demonstrated compliance to an agreed and optimised treatment plan (including high-dose ICS) but have blood eosinophil counts

≥ 300 cells/microlitre (previous 12 months), have had ≥ 4 exacerbations requiring systemic corticosteroids (previous 12 months) or required continuous oral corticosteroids (≥ 5 mg prednisolone or equivalent) for the previous 6 months[NICE]. Similar criteria apply for Reslizumab 3 mg/kg ivi every 4 wks (eosinophil count ≥ 400 cells/microlitre and ≥ 3 exacerbations requiring systemic corticosteroids)[NICE] and Benralizumab 30 mg sc every 4 wks for first three doses, then 30 mg every 8 wks (eosinophil count ≥ 150 cells/microlitre and ≥ 4 exacerbations requiring systemic corticosteroids in the past 12 months or treatment with continuous oral corticosteroids over the previous 6 months)[NICE]. ☠ Screen for and treat helminth infections prior to therapy ☠.

- *Anti-IL-4 and IL-13 monoclonal antibody* (Dupilumab, DUPIXENT) for severe asthmatics with evidence of persistent Th2 inflammation despite optimum Rx with high-dose ICS or oral corticosteroids. Initially 400 mg or 600 mg[1] sc (delivered as two consecutive doses of 200 or 300 mg sc injections at different sites), followed by 200 or 300 mg every 2 wks. ☠ Screen for and treat helminth infections prior to therapy ☠ [1]if currently treated with oral corticosteroids, co-morbid moderate-to-severe atopic eczema or severe chronic rhinosinusitis with nasal polyps.
- *Macrolides* have anti-inflammatory and immunomodulatory effects. Role is controversial. Use azithromycin 250 mg od po three times/wk (Mon/Wed/Fri). Monitor LFTs, QTc and hearing if prolonged use.
- *Immunosuppressants* (methotrexate, ciclosporin and oral gold) may benefit some patients on continuous oral steroids. Marked variability in response and now rarely used with the advent of biological treatments. Use ONLY in specialised centre.
- *Continuous SC terbutaline infusion* may benefit some. Rarely used. Usual dose 5–15 mg/24 h; using the nebuliser solution (2.5 mg/mL). Make up 2–6 mL terbutaline with normal saline to a total 10 mL, infused over 24 h.
- *Bronchial thermoplasty* is occasionally considered for some poorly controlled patients on optimal therapy.

MANAGING COMORBIDITIES

Good practice to manage commonly associated comorbidities:

Gastro-oesphageal reflux disease (GORD): PPI, e.g. omeprazole 20 mg od po.

Allergic rhinitis: Intranasal steroid, e.g. mometasone 100 micrograms each nostril od (NASONEX) or fluticasone 55 micrograms each nostil od (AVAMYS).

Avoid β-blockers (inc eye drops) when treating other conditions.

EXERCISE-INDUCED ASTHMA (EIA)

Acute bronchoconstriction in response to exercise, often related to histamine release. In practice EIA also encompasses patients with chronic asthma, many of whom experience exercise-induced bronchoconstriction (very common trigger). For most patients, consider regular asthma Rx (inc ICS). If exercise symptoms persist → SABA immediately prior to exercise (15 min) ± a trial of sodium cromoglicate 10 mg (2 puffs) qds or nedocromil sodium 4 mg (2 puffs) qds. Leukotriene receptor antagonists, LABAs, oral $β_2$ agonists or theophylline can also be trialled.

ASTHMA IN PREGNANCY

Asthma control may worsen (1/3rd), improve (1/3rd) or remain unchanged (1/3rd). The risk of harm to the foetus from undertreated asthma outweighs any small risks from Rx. Patients should be counselled to continue Rx. ALWAYS closely monitor theophylline levels. Continue leukotriene receptor antagonists if required (limited safety data). Avoid prostaglandin $F_2α$ (for post-partum bleeding) as this can induce bronchospasm. However, prostaglandin E_2 (for labour induction) can be used safely.

BRONCHIECTASIS

Irreversible and abnormal dilation of the bronchi, associated with chronic airway inflammation. Multiple causes. Diagnosis is clinical (chronic sputum production, cough, SOB, haemoptysis and course crackles) and confirmed by airway dilation ±

bronchial wall thickening on high-resolution CT (HRCT).

Cycle of inflammation: inflammation → mucosal damage and ↓ mucociliary clearance → bacterial invasion → inflammation. Many patients are colonised with bacteria, which perpetuate inflammation. Bacterial eradication is therefore an important Rx. Colonising species often depend on stage/severity of disease; usual order of colonisation with ↑ disease severity = *Staphylococcus aureus*, *Haemophilus influenzae*, *Moraxella catarrhalis* and *PSEUDOMONAS aeruginosa*.

2.3.1 Important causes of bronchiectasis

Idiopathic (significant proportion)
Cystic Fibrosis – Always consider!
Post-infective:
    Pneumonia
    TB
    NTM infection (? cause or consequence)
    Bordetella pertussis (Whooping cough)
ABPA
Immune deficiency:
    Hypogammaglobulinaemia
    Secondary to HIV, CLL or nephrotic syndrome
Mucociliary clearance defects:
    Primary ciliary dyskinesia
    Kartagener's syndrome
    Young's syndrome
Toxic insult from aspiration or inhaled noxious gases or chemicals
Obstructing lesion (usually localised disease), e.g. tumour or foreign body
Associated with a number of conditions:
    RA
    Connective tissue disease (e.g. Sjögren's)
    IBD
    Yellow nail syndrome
    Marfan's syndrome

GENERAL MANAGEMENT

Always treat the underlying cause where possible (e.g. immunoglobulin replacement). Consider: (1) respiratory physiotherapy; postural or autogenic drainage, active cycle of breathing technique and cough augmentation (e.g. with flutter valves or positive pressure devices); (2) exercise (± pulmonary rehabilitation); (3) nutritional advice ± dietician referral and supplementation.

ANTIMICROBIAL TREATMENT

Cornerstone of Rx. **Important:** low threshold for starting antibiotics and think ↑dose and ↑duration with bronchiectasis. Prescribed for: exacerbations, 'optimising' patients, eradicating colonising organisms (esp *PSEUDOMONAS*) or long term for those with severe disease. Vital to perform regular sputum MC&S (inc for AFB/NTM and aspergillus) for surveillance. **NB:** *in vitro* sensitivity does not correlate with *in vivo* sensitivity → ALWAYS base antibiotic choice on likely colonising organism, previous successful courses and closely assess clinical response (using objective measures, inc FEV_1 and CRP). Antibiotics can be administered po, nebulised or iv.

Exacerbation of bronchiectasis: Clinical diagnosis (CRP usually ↑ above patient baseline). Choice of antibiotic (inc po or iv) and length of course depends on potential pathogen, prior sputum culture results (and sensitivities), the severity of illness and current/previous response to treatment (Table 2.2[NICE]). **If *PSEUDOMONAS* suspected (or previously cultured):** use ciprofloxacin 750 mg bd po for 2 wks. If po Rx fails or patient unwell → iv therapy, using ceftazidime 2 g tds iv (often for 2 wks) ± aminoglycoside (e.g. gentamycin or tobramycin) if organism resistant. Alternative anti-pseudomonal antibiotics covered by [Table 2.4 – CF in this section].

Eradication of *PSEUDOMONAS*: *PSEUDOMONAS* associated with poorer outcomes: ↑exacerbations, worse CT appearance and ↑decline in lung function. If isolated on respiratory culture → aggressive antibiotic Rx to eradicate using ciprofloxacin

Table 2.2 Choice of antibiotic for treating acute exacerbations of bronchiectasis[NICE]

Antibiotic[1,2]	Dosage (and duration)
Oral antibiotics: **First choice for empirical treatment in absence of susceptibility data (guided by most recent sputum culture and susceptibilities where possible):**	
Amoxicillin[3]	500 mg tds (7–14 days)[4]
Doxycycline	200 mg (first day) then 100 mg od (7–14 days)[4]
Clarithromycin	500 mg bd (7–14 days)[4]
Oral antibiotics: **Alternative choice (if person at higher risk of treatment failure[5]) for empirical treatment in absence of susceptibility data (guided by most recent sputum culture and susceptibilities where possible):**	
Co-amoxiclav	500/125 mg tds (7–14 days)[4]
Levofloxacin[6]	500 mg od/bd (7–14 days)[4]
Intravenous antibiotics: **First choice (if unable to take oral antibiotics or severely unwell) for empirical treatment in the absence of susceptibility data (guided by most recent sputum culture and susceptibilities where possible)[7]:**	
Co-amoxiclav	1.2 g tds
Pipcracillin with tazobactam	4.5 g tds (↑ if necessary to 4.5 g qds)
Levofloxacin[6]	500 mg od/bd
When current susceptibility data available, choose antibiotics accordingly	

[1] See BNF for appropriateness and dosing in hepatic impairment, RF, pregnancy and breastfeeding.

[2] When receiving antibiotic prophylaxis, chose an antibiotic from a different class.

[3] Amoxicillin is the preferred choice in pregnancy.

[4] Course length based on an assessment of bronchiectasis severity, exacerbation severity, previous culture and susceptibility results, and response to treatment.

[5] Higher risk of treatment failure with repeated courses of antibiotics, previous sputum cultures with resistant or atypical bacteria, or a higher risk of developing complications.

[6] The European Medicines Agency's Pharmacovigilance Risk Assessment Committee recommend restricting fluoroquinolone use (potentially long-lasting and disabling side effects). This includes a recommendation not to use them for mild or moderately severe infections unless other antibiotics cannot be used (October 2018).

[7] Review iv antibiotics by 48 hours and consider stepping down to po antibiotics where possible for a total antibiotic course of 7–14 days.

750 mg bd po for 2 wks. If fails → ceftazidime 2 g tds iv (minimum 2 wks) ± aminoglycoside (e.g. gentamycin or tobramycin). Consider use of long-term inh antibiotics: colistin 2 million units neb bd, or tobramycin (**TOBI, BRAMITOB**) 300 mg neb bd.
Macrolides: Possess antibacterial and immunomodulatory properties. Frequently used for colonised or more severe patients; use azithromycin 250/500 mg od po three times/wk (Mon/Weds/Fri). Monitor hearing, QTc and LFTs. GI side effects are common. ↑risk of NTM infection; avoid/discontinue if cultured.

OTHER TREATMENTS

Airflow obstruction: Trial of inhaled bronchodilator (LABA, LAMA) ± ICS (see Asthma/COPD in this section). **Expectorants:** Chronic, tenacious sputum is a hallmark of bronchiectasis. Trials of carbocisteine 750 mg tds po or regular neb hypertonic saline (7%). Nebulised DNase 2500 units od (Dornase alpha, **PULMOZYME**) can be helpful if other Rx fails. **Reflux:** Treat with Omeprazole 20 mg od po. **Haemoptysis:** See Page 244. **Surgery:** Consider for severe localised disease or haemoptysis. Transplantation occasionally indicated.

CHRONIC COUGH

Cough persisting > 8 wks. Can result from respiratory or 'non-respiratory' pathology. ☠ **Always:** assess for underlying lung disease, *esp. cancer* → CXR is a mandatory investigation ☠. Most cases with a normal CXR result from asthma (page 59), gastroesophageal reflux disease (GORD) or postnasal drip. Management usually involves a trial of Rx, based on the most likely cause, typically 3 months, at optimum dose (and delivery) before assessing response. Investigations (e.g. spirometry, peak flow diary, oesophageal pH monitoring or ENT examination) are helpful if Rx fails or there is diagnostic uncertainty.
Cough-variant asthma: Airway inflammation but frequently with minimal bronchoconstriction. Cough is the major (or only) symptom. It is typically worse with exercise or cold air and diurnal PEFR variation usually seen ('morning dip'). Rx is with high

dose ICS, with pMDI ± spacer to ensure optimum inhaler technique and delivery. A heightened cough reflex is also seen with **eosinophilic bronchitis** (sputum eosinophilia without airway hyperresponsiveness or diurnal variation) → cough and sputum EΦ count ↓s with ICS or prednisolone po.

GORD: Initially trial 3 months of PPI: Omeprazole 40 mg od po ± additional Rx if unable to gain symptomatic control, inc ranitidine 150 mg bd po (or 300 mg on), or domperidone 10 mg tds po. Alginates are also helpful, GAVISCON ADVANCE 5–10 mL with meals and at bedtime. Lifestyle measures are important: avoid caffeine, sleeping with an empty stomach and propped up. If diagnostic uncertainty/Rx failure; consider 24-h ambulatory pH monitoring and oesophageal manometry. Nissen Fundoplication may be required for some patients.

Postnasal drip: Often the result of rhinitis (inflammation of nasal mucosa). Can be perennial (most of year), seasonal, allergic (hay fever), non-allergic or infective. Secretions stimulate cough by nasal drip. **Allergic rhinitis:** Non-sedating antihistamine, e.g. cetirizine 10 mg od po + intranasal steroids. Nasal corticosteroid preparations contain beclometasone (BECONASE), betamethasone (BETNASOL), budesonide (RHINOCORT AQUA), fluticasone (FLIXONASE or AVAMYS), mometasone (NASONEX) or triamcinolone (NASACORT). Consult BNF for individual doses. Nasal steroids should be taken in the 'mecca position' or over the end of a bed. **Non-allergic rhinitis:** Best response to sedating antihistamines (helpful antimuscarinic activity), e.g. chlorphenamine (PIRITON) 4 mg qds po + nasal decongestant ± pseudoephedrine 60 mg tds po.

Antitussives: Any underlying condition should be addressed before prescribing. Other causes such as cardiac failure, mediastinal compression, recurrent aspiration, drugs (commonly ACEI) or habitual/psychogenic cough should first be explored. Also consider referral to specialist cough clinic. Codeine phosphate (inc Linctus) can be helpful, but is constipating. Alternatives include pholcodin or dextromethorphan preparations. Sedative antihistamines can also suppress cough.

CHRONIC OBSTRUCTIVE PULMONARY DISEASE (COPD)

Chronic obstructive pulmonary disease (COPD) is a progressive inflammatory condition, characterised by chronic airflow obstruction with minimal or no reversibility. Pathognomonic features are chronic bronchitis, small airway inflammation with fibrosis, and emphysema. Most frequently the result of cigarette smoking but genetic (α_1-antitrypsin), environmental and occupational factors (dusts, chemicals, air pollution and biomass fuel) all play important roles. Diagnosis is based on a history of exposure to risk factors (usually smoking) + evidence of airflow obstruction on spirometry and flow-volume loops (FEV_1:FVC ratio < 0.7 or LLN). It is largely differentiated from asthma on the basis of irreversibility to bronchodilators. However, patients can occasionally display features of both or have both conditions (e.g. Asthma-COPD Overlap Syndrome, or ACOS). The clinical course of COPD is often punctuated with periods of ↑ Sx, otherwise known as exacerbations. Exacerbations are commonly the result of infection (viral or bacterial).

2.5.1 Comprehensive classification of COPD severity. Adapted from Global Initiative for Chronic Obstructive Lung Disease (GOLD) 2020

Any assessment must consider the severity of Sx, spirometry and exacerbation risk:

1 **Confirm fixed airflow obstruction:** A post-bronchodilator FEV_1/FVC < 0.7 (or LLN) is required in the presence of appropriate symptoms and risk factors (e.g. smoking).
2 **Classify the severity of airflow obstruction:** Graded according to the following criteria:

GOLD 1	Mild	$FEV_1 \geq 80\%$ predicted
GOLD 2	Moderate	FEV_1 50–79% predicted
GOLD 3	Severe	FEV_1 30–49% predicted
GOLD 4	Very severe	$FEV_1 < 30\%$ predicted

3 **Assess symptoms:** Using measures of SOB (**modified British Medical Research Council [mMRC] questionnaire**) and quality of life (**COPD Assessment Test [CAT]**).
4 **Assess risk of exacerbation:** Patients can exacerbate frequently (≥ 2/yr) or infrequently, and exacerbations can be managed at home or require hospital admission.

> **Combined assessment:** Categorise each patient as both the GOLD spirometric classification (discussed earlier) and the group (discussed hereunder), e.g. FEV$_1$ = 52%, mMRC = 2 & 3 exacerbations in the last year would be GOLD 2, Group D.

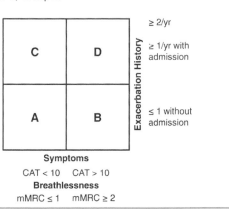

C	D	≥ 2/yr
		≥ 1/yr with admission
A	B	≤ 1 without admission

Exacerbation History

Symptoms

CAT < 10   CAT > 10

Breathlessness

mMRC ≤ 1   mMRC ≥ 2

NON-PHARMACOLOGICAL MANAGEMENT

Smoking cessation is the most important component of Rx (page 229). *Pulmonary rehabilitation* should also be made available to all COPD patients (page 221); an MDT programme with graded exercise and education → ↑exercise tolerance, ↑quality of life and ↓hospital admissions. Consider *nutritional supplementation* for patients with

↓BMI. Assess for anxiety and depression, offering *psychological support* (± antidepressants where appropriate). *Palliative Rx* may be appropriate for severe patients and include breathlessness management techniques (including fan therapy) and opiates.

PHARMACOLOGICAL MANAGEMENT

Aim to ↓symptoms, ↑QoL and ↓ exacerbations. Currently, no Rx (other than smoking cessation) is capable of modifying underlying pathology or ↓mortality. **Vital: always attempt a stepwise therapeutic trial. Stop any medication that has no clinical benefit (after reasonable trial) and monitor Rx compliance and inhaler technique.**

Inhaled treatment

Mainstay of COPD Rx. Options include: *short-acting β_2 agonists (SABA), short-acting muscarinic antagonist (SAMA), long-acting β_2 agonists (LABA), long-acting muscarinic antagonist (LAMA)* and *inhaled corticosteroids (ICS)* (Table 2.3). Multiple combination inhalers are available, including LABA + LAMA, LABA + ICS and LABA + LAMA + ICS triple therapy devices.

All breathless patients should be offered a long-acting bronchodilator (i.e. LAMA ± LABA) to be used regularly, and a SABA (e.g. salbutamol) to be used PRN. SAMAs are available (e.g. ipratropium bromide) but less commonly prescribed. Latest evidence and guidance supports the use of a daily dual LABA + LAMA combination inhaler as the long-acting bronchodilator of choice, wherever possible[GOLD]. However, it may be appropriate to offer LAMA monotherapy for less breathless patients (Figure 2.2).

Unlike asthma, ICS is not a mainstay maintenance treatment for COPD. COPD may be corticosteroid-resistant and ICS use is associated with a greater pneumonia risk in large COPD studies. Therefore, the addition of ICS to LABA + LAMA inhaled treatment is reserved for those patients who are most likely to benefit clinically[GOLD]: (1) hospitalisation(s) for a COPD exacerbation; (2) ≥ 2 exacerbations of COPD per year (despite optimum long-acting bornchodilators); (3) blood eosinophils >

Table 2.3

Long-acting β₂ agonists (LABA)

Salmeterol		
Aerosol		
Non-proprietary	TT BD	e.g. NEOVENT 25 micrograms per metered inhalation
SEREVENT EVOHALER	TT BD	25 micrograms per metered inhalation
SERETIDE EVOHALER (compound; + fluticasone propionate)	TT BD	250/25 micrograms per metered inhalation
Dry powder		
SEREVENT ACCUHALER	T BD	50 micrograms per blister
SERETIDE ACCUHALER (compound; + fluticasone propionate)	T BD	500/50 micrograms per metered inhalation

Formoterol fumarate		
Aerosol		
ATIMOS MODULITE	T BD	12 micrograms per metered inhalation
FOSTAIR (compound; + beclometasone dipropionate)	TT BD	100/6 micrograms per metered inhalation
Dry powder		
Non-proprietary	T BD	e.g. EASYHALER 12 micrograms per metered inhalation
FORADIL	T BD	12 micrograms per capsule
OXIS TURBOHALER	TT BD	6 micrograms per metered inhalation

(Continued)

Table 2.3 (Continued)

SYMBICORT TURBOHALER (compound; + budesonide)	T (400/12) or TT (200/6) BD	200/6 micrograms or 400/12 micrograms per metered inhalation
DUORESP SPIROMAX (compound; + budesonide)	T (320/9) or TT (160/4.5) BD	160/4.5 micrograms & 320/9 micrograms per metered inhalation
FOSTAIR NEXTHALER (compound; + beclometasone dipropionate)	TT BD	100/6 micrograms per metered inhalation
DUALIIR GENUAIR (compound; + aclidinium bromide)	T BD	340/12 micrograms per metered dose
TRIMBOW (compound; + glycopyrronium + beclometasone)	TT BD	87/5/9 micrograms per metered dose
Indacaterol	*Dry powder*	
ONBREZ BREEZHALER	T–TT OD	150 micrograms per capsule
ULTIBRO BREEZHALER (compound; + glycopyrronium)	T OD	85/43 micrograms per capsule
Olodaterol	*Aerosol*	
STRIVERDI RESPIMAT	TT OD	2.5 micrograms per metered dose
SPIOLITO RESPIMAT (compound; + tiotropium)	TT OD	2.5 micrograms per metered dose
Vilanterol	*Dry powder*	
RELVAR ELLIPTA (compound; + fluticasone furoate)	T OD	92/22 & 184/22 micrograms per metered dose
ANORO ELLIPTA (compound; + umeclidinium)	T OD	55/22 micrograms per metered dose

(Continued)

Table 2.3 (Continued)

TRELEGY ELLIPTA (compound; + umeclidinium + fluticasone)	T OD	92/55/22 micrograms per metered dose
Long-acting muscarinic antagonists (LAMA)		
Tiotropium		
Aerosol		
SPIRIVA RESPIMAT	TT OD	2.5 micrograms per metered dose
SPIOLTO RESPIMAT (compound; + olodaterol)	TT OD	2.5 micrograms per metered dose
Dry powder		
SPIRIVA HANDIHALER	T OD	18 micrograms per capsule
Glycopyrronium		
Dry powder		
SEEBRI BREEZHALER	T OD	50 micrograms per capsule
ULTIBRO BREEZHALER (compound; + indacaterol)	T OD	85/43 micrograms per capsule
TRIMBOW (compound; + formoterol + beclometasone)	TT BD	87/5/9 micrograms per metered dose
Aclidinium bromide		
Dry powder		
EKLIRA GENUAIR	T BD	322 micrograms per metered dose
DUAKLIR GENUAIR (compound; + formoterol)	T BD	340/12 micrograms per metered dose
Umeclidinium		
Dry powder		
INCRUSE ELLIPTA	T OD	55 micrograms per metered dose
ANORO ELLIPTA (compound; + vilanterol)	T OD	55/22 micrograms per metered dose
TRELEGY ELLIPTA (compound; + vilanterol + fluticasone)	T OD	92/55/22 micrograms per metered dose

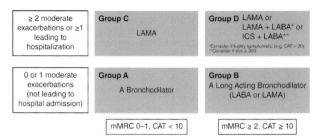

Figure 2.2 Initiating regular inhaled therapy in COPD (From GOLD 2020).

300 cells/µL on FBC; (4) history of asthma, or asthma-like features (e.g. degree of airflow reversibility or atopy) (Figure 2.3). ICS is most commonly prescribed within a LABA + LAMA + ICS triple therapy inhaler, either TRIMBOW (beclomethasone 87 mcg/formoterol 5 mcg/glycopyrronium 9 mcg per metered dose) or TRELEGY ELLIPTA (fluticasone 92 mcg/umeclidinium 55 mcg/vilanterol 22 mcg per metered dose). However, some patients on triple therapy require a higher dose of ICS and are therefore prescribed separate ICS + LABA and LAMA devices.

Any decision to start ICS in COPD should be balanced against the risks of therapy (i.e. local adverse effects, repeated pneumonia and mycobacterial disease). Patients with a peripheral blood eosinophil

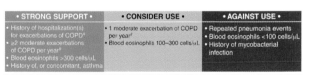

Figure 2.3 Factors to consider when initiating ICS treatment in COPD (From GOLD 2020).

count > 300 cells/µL on FBC are most likely to benefit and those with < 100 cells/µL very unlikely to benefit. ICS should be withdrawn in COPD when it is not indicated or a trial leads to no clinical improvement. ICS monotherapy should never be prescribed in COPD.

Additional treatments

Theophylline: Consider if trial of other bronchodilators is unsuccessful, patient unable to effectively use inhaled Rx or on-going Sx despite maximal inh Rx. Beware toxicity, esp in elderly with comorbidities. **Always specify brand!–** SLO-PHYLLIN 250–500 mg bd po, UNIPHYLLIN CONTINUS 200–400 mg bd po, NEULIN SA (175) 175–350 mg bd po or NEULIN SA (250) 250–500 mg bd po.

Mucolytics: Consider for those with chronic productive coughs, typically carbocisteine (MUCODYNE) 375–750 mg tds po.

Nebulisers: Reserve for patients with poor inhaler technique (inc cognitively impaired) and those with on-going Sx despite maximal inhaled Rx. Can use SABA (salbutamol 2.5 mg PRN) ± SAMA (ipratropium bromide 250–500 micrograms QDS).

Oral glucocorticoids: Long-term use not recommended! If trialled (e.g. asthma component) use ↓ dose and consider osteoporosis prophylaxis.

Azithromycin: Macrolides are immunomodulatory and may be beneficial for patients with recurrent exacerbations. NOT routinely recommended due to concerns over bacterial resistance. Use azithromycin 250–500 mg po/od/three times a wk (Mon/Weds/Fri). Stop Rx if any changes in hearing (e.g. tinnitus), monitor QTc and LFTs. GI side effects are common → discontinue or try reduced dose. ↑risk of NTM; avoid/discontinue if cultured.

Roflumilast: A phosphodiesterase type-4 inhibitor, licensed as an adjunct to bronchodilators for the maintenance Rx of severe COPD associated with chronic bronchitis and a history of frequent exacerbations (≥ 2 exacerbations in last 12 months despite triple inhaled therapy[NICE]. *Dose* = 250 micrograms od po for 28 days then 500 micrograms od.

Vaccination: Pneumococcal and annual influenza vaccinations recommended.

Oxygen: See page 176. Can be prescribed as: *short burst oxygen therapy (SBOT)* for symptomatic relief, e.g. after exertion, *ambulatory oxygen* and/or *long-term oxygen therapy (LTOT)*. LTOT is indicated in all stable patients with PaO_2 < 7.3 kPa, or stable patients with PaO_2 7.3–8 kPa and ≥ 1 of: 2° polycythaemia, nocturnal hypoxaemia (SaO_2 < 90% for > 30% of the time), peripheral oedema or pulmonary hypertension.

Cor pulmonale: Right ventricular failure in response to ↑ pulmonary vascular resistance; may require diuretic therapy to manage oedema. Should prompt O_2 assessment.

FURTHER INTERVENTION

Surgery: Ventilation and Sx can be improved in some patients with upper lobe-predominant emphysema or large bullae by *lung volume reduction surgery (LVRS)* or *bullectomy*, respectively. *Endoscopically sited valves or coils* can achieve similar results in selected patients. *Lung transplantation* is occasionally suitable.

Domiciliary non-invasive ventilation (NIV): may be appropriate for selected patients with chronic hypercapnic type 2 ✖; usually administered nocturnally. See page 204.

CYSTIC FIBROSIS

Multi-system disease resulting from a mutation in the gene encoding for the cystic fibrosis transmembrane conductance regulator (CFTR; a chloride channel). Defective CFTR → dysregulation of salt and water movement across membranes → viscous secretions in multiple organs (e.g. lungs or pancreas). Viscous lung secretions become colonised with pathogenic bacteria and the subsequent inflammatory response is responsible for lung damage and irreversible bronchiectasis. Dx is based on the recognition of clinical features, a positive sweat test (confirmed > 60 mmol/L Cl⁻; equivocal 30–60 mmol/L Cl⁻) and

---

2.6.1 Genetics of cystic fibrosis

- Autosomal recessive
- Gene on long arm of chromosome 7
- One in 25 Caucasians carry gene; 1 in 2500 UK live births have CF
- > 1700 different mutations are recognised
- Commonest mutation is ΔF508 (approximately 70% of CF cases in Europe)
- Five other mutations typically occur at a frequency > 1%: G542X, G551D, W1282X, N1303K and R553X
- Different mutations may be associated with a specific clinical phenotype

Most patients are Dx as neonates or children (screening or compatible clinical findings).

---

genetic testing (Box 2.6.1). **NB:** genetic testing is NOT available for all known mutations and some mutations may NOT be sufficient for Dx. In a small proportion, CF is difficult to Dx with certainty. These patients can be described as 'CF unlikely', 'non-classic CF' or 'CFTR-related disorder'. In equivocal cases, transepithelial nasal potential difference can be measured. Neonatal screening is performed in the UK.

GENERAL PRINCIPLES OF MANAGEMENT

Although gene therapy trials are currently on-going, there remains no cure for CF. Mutation-specific therapies are available however, e.g. Ivacaftor for G551D mutation (only ≈ 4% of patients worldwide). All patients are managed in CF centres which provide MDT care (physicians, specialist nurses, physiotherapists, dieticians, pharmacists and psychologists). Compliance with Rx can be problematic, esp with adolescents. **NB:** drug pharmacokinetics are different in cystic fibrosis with ↑volume of distribution, ↓plasma concentration and ↑elimination (renal and non-renal) → many drugs require different dosing, including antibiotics (discussed hereunder).

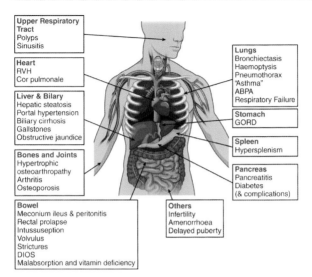

Upper Respiratory Tract
Polyps
Sinusitis

Heart
RVH
Cor pulmonale

Liver & Bilary
Hepatic steatosis
Portal hypertension
Biliary cirrhosis
Gallstones
Obstructive jaundice

Bones and Joints
Hypertrophic osteoarthropathy
Arthritis
Osteoporosis

Bowel
Meconium ileus & peritonitis
Rectal prolapse
Intussuseption
Volvulus
Strictures
DIOS
Malabsorption and vitamin deficiency

Lungs
Bronchiectasis
Haemoptysis
Pneumothorax
"Asthma"
ABPA
Respiratory Failure

Stomach
GORD

Spleen
Hypersplenism

Pancreas
Pancreatitis
Diabetes
(& complications)

Others
Infertility
Amenorrhoea
Delayed puberty

Figure 2.4 CF manifestations.

TREATING CF BRONCHIECTASIS

The focus of Rx is to maintain lung function. This is primarily done by targeting the pathogenic bacteria that colonise the airways, using antimicrobials. These bacteria play an important role in the pathogenesis of bronchiectasis. Colonisation occurs from an early age and changes as the patient grows older (Figure 2.5). They may also become ↑ resistant. When organism levels rise, this will manifest clinically as an 'exacerbation' (↑sputum, ↑T°, lethargy, ↑SOB, ↑CRP and ↓FEV$_1$ are all good indicators). Both colonisation and exacerbations should be Rx aggressively (as follows).

Antimicrobials

Cornerstone of Rx. Important: Low threshold for starting, ↑dose and ↑duration of Rx (usually 2–3 wks). Prescribed for

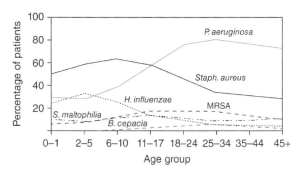

Figure 2.5 Chronic bacterial colonisation and infection in CF.

exacerbations, 'optimising' patients, eradicating colonising
organisms (esp *PSEUDOMONAS*) or for long term in those with
severe disease. Vital to perform regular sputum MC&S (inc for
AFB and aspergillus) for surveillance. **NB:** *in vitro* sensitivity does
NOT correlate with *in vivo* sensitivity → ALWAYS base antibiotic
choice on likely colonising organism, previous successful courses
and closely assess the clinical response (using objective measures,
inc FEV$_1$ and CRP). **If** *PSEUDOMONAS* **has been previously
isolated:** ensure it is adequately covered with current antibiotic
choice. Antibiotics for CF can be administered po, nebulised or
iv. Rx can be as an inpatient (unwell) or as an outpatient. Patients
can have midlines, PICCs or Port-a-caths inserted to allow iv
antibiotics to be administered at home. ☠ ALWAYS ensure the
first dose of any iv antibiotic is administered in hospital, even if
previously prescribed, as allergy, sensitisation and cross-reactivity
are much more common in CF! ☠ **NB:** antibiotic resistance is a
major problem, esp with β-lactams and repeated courses. ALWAYS
consult local policies and microbiology.
Staphylococcus aureus: Important colonising organism.
Attempt eradication even if patient is asymptomatic. Use

flucloxacillin 1–2 g qds po/iv min. 2 wks. If penicillin resistance or allergy use erythromycin 500 mg bd po.

Haemophilus influenzae: If isolated, Rx is usually with amoxicillin 500 mg–1 g tds po/iv *or* co-amoxiclav 625 mg tds po (1.2 g tds iv). Min. Rx is 2 wks.

PSEUDOMONAS aeruginosa: Ubiquitous Gram-negative pathogen, which is intrinsically resistant to multiple antibiotics (multiple efflux systems and can form biofilms). It is associated with poorer outcomes in CF. **Important:** the first isolate of a non-mucoid *PSEUDOMONAS* should be Rx promptly and aggressively, even if patient asymptomatic. **Eradication:** always consult local policies which may vary. *Typical regimen:* ciprofloxacin 750 mg bd po (min. 1 month) with neb colistin 1–2 million units bd (3 months). If successfully eradicated but a subsequent new isolate is found → reattempt eradication. If eradication fails or the patient is unwell → trial of iv therapy with two anti-pseudomonals, e.g. ceftazidime 2 g tds iv (min. 2 wks) + aminoglycoside (e.g. gentamycin or tobramycin) followed by the longer-term use of an inh antibiotic, usually tobramycin (TOBI, BRAMITOB) 300 mg nebulised bd. **Exacerbations:** can be treated with po or iv antibiotics, depending on severity. *Mild exacerbation* – Use ciprofloxacin 750 mg bd po; *severe exacerbation* – Base choice of iv on previous successfully regimens and culture sensitivities, and use two antibiotics which work synergistically (normally β-lactam + aminoglycoside) for 10–14 days. *Typical iv regimen:* ceftazidime 2 g tds iv + tobramycin 7 mg/kg od iv. ☠ ALWAYS consider renal function with aminoglycosides and avoid if GFR < 20 mL/min. Stop if any dizziness or balance disturbance ☠.

Burkholderia cepacia: Complex of 11 species that form biofilms and are highly resistant (very poor prognosis). Microbiology advice is recommended! Eradication following an initial isolate is often attempted: ceftazidime 2 g tds iv + tobramycin 7 mg/kg od iv. This is often followed up with chronic suppressive nebulised antibiotics: tobramycin (TOBI, BRAMITOB) 300 mg bd, *or* ceftazidime 1 g bd *or* meropenem 250 mg bd.

Table 2.4 Examples of common iv antibiotics used to treat *PSEUDOMONAS*

Drug	Class	Dose	Additional information
Amikacin	Aminoglycoside	15 mg/kg od (↓ to 12 mg/kg od if GFR < 20 mL/min)	Follow local guidance for peak and trough level measurement
Aztreonam	β-Lactam	2 g tds	↓if GFR < 30 mL/min
Ceftazidime	β-Lactam	2 g tds	Monitor LFTs if liver disease ↓if GFR < 15 mL/min
Ciprofloxacin	Fluoroquinolone	400 mg bd	po preferable ↓if GFR < 10 mL/min
Colistimethate sodium (colistin, COLOMYCIN)	Polymyxin	2 million units tds	↓if GFR < 20 mL/min
Meropenem	β-Lactam	2 g tds	Monitor LFTs ↓if GFR < 20 mL/min
Piperacillin/ tazobactam (TAZOCIN)	β-Lactam	4.5 g tds	Monitor LFTs ↓if GFR < 20 mL/min
Ticarcillin/ clavulanic acid (TIMENTIN)	β-Lactam	3.2 g qds	Monitor LFTs ↓if GFR < 30 mL/min
Tobramycin	Aminoglycoside	7 mg/kg od (↓ to 3 mg/kg od if GFR < 50 mL/min; avoid if < 20 mL/min)	Follow local guidance for peak and trough level measurement

MRSA: Confers worsening lung function. Eradication often attempted, e.g. rifampicin 600 mg bd po (450 mg if < 50 kg) + fusidic acid 500 mg–1 g tds po. If patient is unwell or lung function deteriorating → vancomycin 1 g bd iv.

Stenotrophomonas maltophilia: Not always associated with ↑ Sx or ↓lung function and Rx not always required. Use co-trimoxazole 960 mg bd po.

Macrolides: Possess immunomodulatory and antibacterial effects → ↑ FEV$_1$ and ↓ need for iv antibiotics. Use azithromycin 500 mg po (250 mg if < 40 kg) od three times a wk (usually Mon, Weds and Fri). Stop Rx if any changes in hearing (e.g. tinnitus), monitor QTc and LFTs. GI side effects are common → discontinue or try ↓ dose. ↑risk of NTM; avoid/discontinue if cultured.

Other drugs and management considerations

Physiotherapy: Vital component of CF Rx. Several chest physiotherapy techniques are used: active cycle of breathing control, autogenic drainage, percussion, flutter devices, positive pressure masks and oscillation vests.

Recombinant DNase (RhDNase – PULMOZYME): ↓ sputum viscosity by cleaving dead NΦ-derived DNA. ↑ FEV$_1$ and ↓ exacerbations and may ↑ survival. Start with objective evidence of sputum retention (e.g. ↓FEV$_1$ or small airway disease). Use 2.5 mg (2500 units) neb daily. Continue after 3-month trial if any objective evidence of improvement.

Hypertonic saline: 7% saline (NEBUSAL 4 mL nebule) is nebulised as adjunct to physiotherapy to aid sputum clearance. ☠ May induce bronchoconstriction; initially use ↓ dose in those with airflow obstruction and administer first dose in hospital, performing pre- and post-spirometry ☠.

Mannitol (BRONCHITOL): Osmotic agent which may ↑ sputum clearance. Use only if no improvement/intolerance to RhDNase or hypertonic saline^{NICE}. Maintenance dose = 400 mg neb bd 5–15 mins after bronchodilator.

Allergic Bronchopulmonary Aspergillosis (ABPA): Not uncommon in CF. Maintain high index of suspicion. Rx as per ABPA in asthma (page 55) using prednisolone + itraconazole 200 mg po bd (works as a steroid sparing agent). Voriconazole 200 mg bd po (400 mg day 1; half the dose if < 40 kg) or posaconazole 400 mg bd are alternative second- or third-line agents.

Haemoptysis: Minor haemoptysis is common in CF, esp with infection. Major haemoptysis can be life-threatening (page 244).
Pneumothorax: Common in older patients with severe lung disease. Very low threshold for chest drain insertion. Persistent air leaks are frequent and may require prolonged drainage and suction. Cardiothoracic referral and discussion with patient's transplant centre should be considered. ☠ Avoid pleurodesis in transplant candidates ☠.
Non-tuberculous mycobacteria: ↑ prevalent in CF. Significance often unclear. Persistent culture in patients with declining lung function should prompt a consideration of Rx (page 145).
'CF asthma': Many CF patients exhibit asthma-like symptoms and bronchial hyper-reactivity. Rx as per standard asthma stepwise approach (page 59).

TREATING COMMON NON-PULMONARY MANIFESTATIONS

Nutrition: Maintaining a BMI > 20 is problematic with severe disease and infection. ↑ protein and calorific diets are advised. Supplemental feeding (nasogastric or gastrostomy) is commonly required. A major factor is pancreatic insufficiency → CREON (lipase, protease and amylase) 10,000, 25,000, 40,000 capsules can be taken pre-meals and adjusted according to meal content to control steatorrhoea and prevent energy loss. Specialist CF dietician advice is important. *Typical starting regimen:* 1–2 capsules (10,000 CREON) with each meal and 1 capsule with fat-containing snacks. Fat soluble vitamins (A, D, E & K) are malabsorbed and should also be replaced.
Distal Intestinal Obstructive Syndrome (DIOS): Intestinal obstruction 2° to thickened stool (meconium ileus equivalent). Rarely requires surgery and can be managed medically. Check enzyme supplementation (poor compliance can be a cause), ensure adequate hydration and commence osmotic laxatives (e.g. lactulose 5–20 mL bd ± MOVICOL 1–2 sachets bd). Gastrografin is highly osmotic and can also be used orally (100 mL in 400 mL water), rectally (100 mL bd) or instilled at the site of the obstruction by

colonoscopy. Intestinal lavage with Kleen Prep, via nasogastric tube is occasionally required.

Reflux: More common in CF than general population. Rx with omeprazole 20–40 mg po od.

CF-related diabetes (CFRD): Common complication of CF. Requires insulin and CANNOT be Rx with oral hypoglycaemics. The dietary restriction of sugar is also NOT advocated. Diabetic ketoacidosis (DKA) is exceptionally rare in CFRD and is managed conventionally.

Osteoporosis: Multifactorial aetiology (e.g. vitamin D deficiency, ↓ activity, steroid use, delayed puberty). Rx is with calcium and vitamin D supplementation (e.g. ADCAL D₃), weight-bearing exercise, hormones for delayed puberty ± bisphosphonate (e.g. alendronic acid).

Hepatobiliary disease: Wide spectrum including steatosis (fatty liver), cirrhosis, gallstones and cholecystitis. Regular ultrasound and LFTs (inc prothrombin time) are required. ALWAYS take care when starting new medication in a CF patient with liver disease (esp antibiotics, antifungals and NSAIDs). Ursodeoxycholic acid (12 mg/kg daily) is often used to improve bile flow and vitamin K replaced when prothrombin time is prolonged. Complications are otherwise managed in conjunction with gastroenterology. Some patients require liver transplantation.

Nasal polyps and sinusitis: Very common manifestation of CF. Initial Rx with nasal steroids but surgical intervention may be required.

OTHER ISSUES

Pregnancy: CF men are infertile and women subfertile. Encourage women to discuss reproductive plans. Pregnancy with ↓lung function can compromise maternal and foetal health.

Genetic counselling and screening: Offer to all CF patients and partners.

Palliative care: Emphasis should be placed on managing symptoms when it is acknowledged by the team that further active treatment would be futile.

Lung transplantation: May be appropriate for some CF patients; assessment at transplant centre.

Gene therapy: Large clinical trials currently in progress.

MUTATION-SPECIFIC TREATMENTS

CFTR modulators are available. NHS England commissions **Ivacaftor** (KALYDECO) 150 mg po bd for CF patients with the specific G551D mutation or one of these gating (class III) mutations: G551D, G1244E, G1349D, G178R, G551S, S1251N, S1255P, S549N or S549R. Genotyping is required before starting Rx and the patient must have the mutation in at least one allele of the CFTR gene. Ivacaftor is a CFTR potentiator (allows the defective channel to open and pass chloride ions). In responsive patients it normalises sweat sodium, ↑lung function, ↑BMI and ↓exacerbation frequency. NHS England also commissions: (1) Lumacaftor with Ivacaftor (ORKAMBI) 400/250 mg po bd for CF patients who are homozygous for the F508del mutation; (2) Tezacaftor with ivacaftor (SYMKEVI) 100/150 mg po od (with Ivacaftor 150 mg taken separately in the evening) for CF patients who are homozygous for the F508del mutation or heterozygous in the CFTR gene for any one of 14 mutations (P67L, R117C, L206W, R352Q, A455E, D579G, 711+3A→G, S945L, S977F, R1070W, D1152H, 2789+5G→A, 3272-26A→G, and 3849+10kbC→T) combined with the F508del mutation; (3) Tezacaftor with ivacaftor and elexacaftor (**KAFTRIO**) 50/75/100 mg (two tablets po od with Ivacaftor 150 mg taken separately in the evening) for CF patients who are homozygous for the F508del mutation or heterozygous for the F508del mutation with any other mutation.

INTERSTITIAL LUNG DISEASE

Group of conditions characterised by diffuse parenchymal/interstitial inflammation and fibrosis of unknown aetiology (aka idiopathic interstitial pneumonia). Pathogenesis is poorly understood. Current classification identifies seven distinct subtypes (Table 2.5; in order of frequency). Commonest

Table 2.5

	Important clinical features	Important HRCT features	Histology	Specific treatment/ Prognosis
Idiopathic pulmonary fibrosis (IPF)	Older (> 60 yrs) *Onset:* months – yrs SOB, cough, fine basal late inspiratory crackles, clubbing (≈ 50%), ↓PO$_2$ and cor pulmonale (later).	Fibrosis and honeycombing in a subpleural and basal distribution, traction bronchiectasis, minimal ground glass (if extensive consider alternative diagnosis).	*Usual interstitial pneumonia (UIP)* – patchy interstitial fibrosis with alternating areas of normal lung. Displays temporal heterogeneity with scattered fibroblastic foci, dense acellular collagen and architectural changes (honeycomb). Minimal inflammation.	*Options include:* (1) Supportive Rx (below); (2) Trial of drug monotherapy (below); (3) Lung transplantation (< 65 yrs old). Prognosis poor.
Non-specific interstitial pneumonia (NSIP)	Younger (40–50 yrs) Onset: months–yrs Associations: connective tissue disease, drugs, infection and immunodeficiency (inc. HIV).	Fine reticulation with ground glass (often basal predominant). Honeycombing is rare.	Uniform interstitial inflammation and fibrosis (cannot be classified into one of the other subtypes).	Oral prednisolone (usually 0.5 mg/kg od); consider additional immuno-suppression if patient fails to respond. Prognosis usually good (stable or improve on Rx).

(Continued)

Table 2.5 (*Continued*)

	Important clinical features	Important HRCT features	Histology	Specific treatment/ Prognosis
Cryptogenic organising pneumonia (COP)	Younger (mean 55 yrs) Onset: months Systemic features: malaise, ↑T°, wt loss. Think 'slow to resolve' pneumonia/ LRTI Associated with RA.	Patchy consolidation in a subpleural and peribronchial distribution.	Plugging of alveolar spaces (± bronchioles) with granulation tissue. No architectural distortion.	Oral prednisolone (usually 1 mg/kg od) ± pulsed iv methylprednisolone (750 mg–1 g for first 3 days); consider additional immunosuppression if fail to respond or critically unwell, usually cyclophosphamide. Prognosis good (improve within days).
Acute interstitial pneumonia (AIP)	Any age. Onset: rapid days to wks (often resembles pneumonia or viral illness with subsequent ARDS).	Patchy consolidation with diffuse symmetrical and bilateral ground glass.	Diffuse alveolar change with oedema, hyaline membranes and fibroblast proliferation; biopsy often required to differentiate from ARDS.	Typically require high flow O₂, ITU admission and ventilation. Try pulsed iv methylprednisolone (750 mg–1 g for first 3 days) followed by oral prednisolone (usually 1 mg/kg od). Prognosis very poor (50% mortality).

(*Continued*)

Table 2.5 (*Continued*)

	Important clinical features	Important HRCT features	Histology	Specific treatment/ Prognosis
Respiratory bronchiolitis- associated interstitial lung disease (RB-ILD)	Younger (30–40 yrs) Cigarette smokers (pack yrs > 30). Mild Sxs. Onset: over yrs.	Ill-defined centrilobular nodules, ground glass and bronchial wall thickening (and associated with centrilobular emphysema).	Pigmented macrophages in bronchioles.	Smoking cessation. Oral prednisolone occasionally required. Prognosis very good.
Desquamative interstitial pneumonia (DIP)	Younger; considered more severe form of RB-ILD. Smokers (or dust inhalation). Onset: wks to months. Clubbing is common.	Diffuse ground glass.	Pigmented macrophages in alveoli.	Smoking cessation. Oral prednisolone occasionally required. Prognosis very good (may relapse-remit).
Lymphoid interstitial pneumonia (LIP)	Any age. Onset: yrs. Usually associated with: connective tissue disease (Sjögren's, RA, SLE), immunodeficiency, infection, autoimmune disease (e.g. haemolytic/ pernicious anaemia, Hashimoto's, PBC, MG) or some drugs (e.g. phenytoin).	Diffuse ground glass, often with reticulation and cysts. Honeycombing sometimes seen.	Diffuse interstitial lymphoid infiltrates (difficult to distinguish from lymphoma).	Oral prednisolone (usually 0.5–1 mg/kg od). Consider additional immunosuppression if fail to respond. Prognosis variable (progression with extensive fibrosis in 1/3rd).

is idiopathic pulmonary fibrosis (IPF; previously termed cryptogenic fibrosis alveolitis). IPF is also considered separately hereunder.

A fibrotic process is usually apparent from the Hx, examination, CXR and lung function (restrictive pattern ± ↓gas transfer). However, a specific IPF diagnosis often requires an **MDT approach**; taking into account clinical features, HRCT findings and histology (most specific). Histological samples can be obtained by surgical or transbronchial biopsy (**NB**: patchy processes may not be seen; therefore target most diseased lobes at bronchoscopy). Not all patients are suitable for biopsy and CT imaging and the recognition of patterns has improved. Therefore, it is now common practice to reserve biopsy for where diagnostic doubt remains after HRCT (esp if this could/might alter the Rx).

IDIOPATHIC PULMONARY FIBROSIS (IPF)

Commonest idiopathic ILD ($\approx$ 200/100,000 of > 75 yr olds). Suspect in older patients with cough and SOB over several months + other classical features: hypoxia (at rest or desaturating on exercise), fine basal late inspiratory crackles, clubbing, signs of cor pulmonale, restrictive pattern on lung function (↓lung volumes ± ↓gas transfer) and CXR changes (reticular; either extensive or in a peripheral and basal pattern). **Diagnosis:** from clinical and HRCT findings (Table 2.5) ± biopsy. Biopsy (via VATS or thoracotomy) is reserved for diagnostic uncertainty (e.g. younger patients, ground glass change). *Histology* = UIP (can be seen with other conditions, e.g. connective tissue disease or asbestosis). **Prognosis:** generally poor (mean survival = 3–5 yrs) but course can be variable and difficult to predict; some remain stable for years, others rapidly decline after relative stability.

Management

Treatment should be patient-specific and in the context of severity, projected disease course, existing comorbidity and patient wishes.

The 'typically poor but highly variable prognosis' and unpredictable efficacy of Rx should be explained.

Disease monitoring: Assess Sx and perform regular lung function (↓ FVC/TLCO by 10–15% are significant). *Remember:* Rx may not ↑lung function but stabilise/slow rate of progression. Some patients (e.g. the less symptomatic) may benefit from a 'watch-and-wait' approach.

Pharmacotherapy: Very limited. Several are now NO longer recommended and may be in fact be harmful, i.e. corticosteroid monotherapy (except with exacerbation or diagnostic uncertainty, e.g. some ground glass on HRCT), 'triple therapy' (prednisolone, azathioprine and N-acetylcysteine) and anticoagulation with warfarin. Monotherapy with *N-acetylcysteine* 600 mg po tds is still used (anti-oxidant/anti-fibrotic). *Pirfenidone* (ESBRIET) and *Nintedanib* (OFEV) are now licensed (see Box); pirfenidone maintenance dose = 801 mg (three capsules) po tds (initially titrate as 1 capsule tds for 1 wk then 2 capsules tds for 1 wk), nintedanib maintenance dose = 150 mg po bd. Often limited by SE and regular monitoring required. Consider suitable patients for clinical trials through local centres!

2.7.1 Pirfenidone and nintedanib for IPF[NICE]

- Recommended as options for treating IPF if FVC > 50% and < 80% predicted.
- Discontinue if evidence of disease progression; defined as ↓predicted FVC ≥ 10% within any 12-month period.

Supportive care: Consider home O_2 (page 176) and PR (page 221). GORD is common and may play a role in pathogenesis (use PPI; omeprazole 20 mg po od). Palliative measures appropriate for advanced disease (page 114).

Lung transplantation: See page 110. Consider for: younger symptomatic patients (< 65 yrs) with TLCO < 40%, confirmed diagnosis (UIP histology), ↓FVC ≥ 10% over 6 months, desaturation on 6MWT and honeycombing on HRCT.

2.7.2 Acute exacerbations of IPF

- Exacerbation of Sx, usually over several days to wks.
- Aetiology may be unclear or 2° to infection, LVF or PE (common in IPF).
- CXR usually shows ↑shadowing from baseline (often ground glass on HRCT).

MANAGEMENT

1 Consider antibiotics if infection suspected (± BAL if an atypical infection suspected, e.g. PCP; patients are usually too hypoxic for bronchoscopy!)
2 Corticosteroids, either prednisolone 0.5–1 mg/kg/od *or* methylprednisolone 750 mg–1 g iv for 3 days first followed by po prednisolone. **NB:** always cover steroids with broad spectrum antibiotics.

COVID-19

Coronavirus (COVID-19) infection results in severe acute respiratory syndrome coronavirus 2 (SARS-CoV-2). Responsible for worldwide pandemic in 2019–2020. Acute infection causes pneumonitis with respiratory failure in a proportion of patient. Limited trial data/no consensus for optimum management but many centres using corticosteroids (e.g. dexamethasone or mehtylprednsiolone) acutely. Interstitial lung disease is an increasingly recognised complication in survivors, mainly organising pneumonia. No consensus for management but many centres treating with corticosteroids (e.g. prednisolone).

HYPERSENSITIVITY PNEUMONITIS

Group of conditions caused by the inhalation of an Ag to which the patient is sensitised → alveolar inflammation. Previously known as Extrinsic Allergic Alveolitis (EAA). Can be *acute* (short exposure to ↑Ag concentrations; reversible) or *chronic/subacute* (long-term exposure to ↓ concentrations; less reversible or irreversible with fibrosis). Involves type IV (T-cell-mediated with granuloma formation) and/or type III hypersensitivity (Ab-Ag immune complex formation). NOT type I (Eφ- and IgE-mediated). **Causes:** Many different Ags (mostly organic) are recognised. Some important examples are listed in Table 2.6.

Table 2.6 Causes of hypersensitivity pneumonitis

Disease	Exposure	Major Ag
Bird fancier's lung	Avian proteins	Feathers, bird droppings
Bagassosis	Mouldy sugar cane	*Thermophilic actinomycetes*
Cheese washer's lung	Cheese mould	*Penicillium casei*
Chemical worker's lung (Isocyanate HP)	Paints, resins and polyurethane foams	Toluene diisocyanate, Hexamethylene diisocyanate or Methylene bisphenyl isocyanate
Compost lung	Compost	*Aspergillus spp*
Farmer's lung	Mouldy hay	*Thermophilic actinomycetes, Aspergillus spp, Saccharopolyspora rectivirgula* or *Micropolyspora faeni*
Hot tub lung	Hot tub mists	*Mycobacterium avium* complex
Humidifier (or air-conditioner) lung	Contaminated systems	Bacteria (*Thermoactinomyces candidus, Bacillus subtilis, Bacillus cereus, Klebsiella oxytoca, Thermophilic actinomycetes*), fungi (*Aureobasidium pullulans*) and amoebae (*Naegleria gruberi, Acanthamoeba polyhaga, Acanthamoeba castellani*)
Japanese summer house HP	Damp wood, mats, dusts	*Trichosporon cutaneum*
Malt worker's lung	Mouldy barley	*Aspergillus clavatus*
Mushroom worker's lung	Mushroom compost	Thermophilic actinomycetes
Rat lung	Rat proteins	Rat droppings
Shell lung	Mollusc shells	Mollusc shell proteins

CLINICAL FEATURES

Acute HP: Cough, $\uparrow$T°, SOB $\pm$ wheeze within a few hours of exposure. **Chronic HP:** progressive SOB, cough $\pm$ Wt loss over months to years.

INVESTIGATIONS

Diagnosis usually based on Hx of Ag exposure + typical clinical features + supportive investigations (i.e. CXR, HRCT, lung fx, bloods; see Box). Some cases require bronchoscopy + BAL ($\uparrow$lymphocytes) *or* lung biopsy (transbronchial or surgical).

2.8.1 Investigations in hypersensitivity pneumonitis

CXR: Acute HP: Diffuse infiltrates/nodules or ground-glass change; *chronic HP* – $\downarrow$lung volumes with reticulation.

HRCT: Acute HP: Diffuse ground-glass change with micronodules and mosaic attenuation (air trapping; may require expiratory scan); *chronic HP* – addition of fibrosis (e.g. honeycomb change and traction bronchiectasis).

Lung function: Restrictive with $\downarrow$gas transfer (obstruction may also be present)

Blood tests: $\uparrow$NΦ/$\uparrow$CRP/$\uparrow$serum precipitins (IgG)

MANAGEMENT

Most importantly: strict allergen avoidance *or* $\downarrow$exposure (respiratory protection, $\uparrow$ventilation or air filters) $\rightarrow$ resolution of Sx (acute HS). Corticosteroids, i.e. prednisolone 0.5 mg/kg po od are occasionally used (usually acutely; less effective in chronic HP) until Sx and radiological changes improve (some patients require maintenance Rx at a lower dose). Excellent prognosis for acute HP with allergen avoidance. However, chronic HP is much more likely to develop with chronic ✖, cor pulmonale and eventual death.

LUNG CANCER

Common 1° tumour in both men and women. Usually smoking related (>90%); other risk factors include asbestos, pulmonary fibrosis, radiation and heavy metal exposure. Classified according to histology (see Box); **non-small cell lung cancer (NSCLC)** and **small cell lung cancer (SCLC)** most important.

May be asymptomatic (incidental CXR/CT) *or* present with Sxs and signs from the tumour itself (e.g. cough, SOB, haemoptysis, dysphagia, stridor), metastasis/local invasion (e.g. chest pain, effusion, liver/bone pain, lymphadenopathy, hoarse voice, neurological, $\uparrow Ca^{2+}$, lymphangitis carcinomatosis) or paraneoplastic syndromes (e.g. cachexia, clubbing, HPOA, SIADH, Cushing's, cerebellar syndrome, Lambert-Eaton myasthenic

---

2.9.1 Lung cancer classification

Non-small cell lung cancer (NSCLC) ≈ **80%**

    Squamous cell carcinoma

        Most common

        Can be multiple and cavitate

    Adenocarcinoma

        Most common in 'never smokers' and as metastatic disease from other sites

    Bronchoalveolar cell carcinoma (BAC)

        Now reclassified as subtype of adenocarcinoma

Small cell lung cancer (SCLC) ≈ **15%**

        Most aggressive and usually extensively metastasised at presentation (median survival 6 wks)

Others

        Including large cell carcinoma, adenosquamous carcinoma, carcinoid tumours, sarcomatoid carcinoma, salivary gland tumours, pre-invasive lesions.

syndrome, dermatomyositis, limbic encephalitis). ☠ **Always look out for signs of common oncological emergencies: SVCO, cord compression, ↑Ca^{2+}, SIADH, massive haemoptysis or upper airway obstruction (page 269)** ☠. *Pancoast's tumours* (apical) can damage the sympathetic chain to cause Horner's syndrome (miosis, ptosis, enophthalmos, anhydrosis) or invade the brachial plexus.

Important: Smokers/ex-smokers > 50 yrs with any chest Sx should always have a CXR (± further investigations, e.g. CT)!

INVESTIGATIONS

Any suspected lung cancer is referred under the '2-week wait' (i.e. 14 days to first appointment). The aim is to obtain histological diagnosis, stage the cancer and offer treatment promptly (≤ 62 days from referral or ≤ 31 days from decision to treat). Diagnosis and staging (below) is achieved in fewest possible tests/ procedures, e.g. biopsy of metastasis will simultaneously give diagnosis and staging. Patient care is determined by an MDT, which includes a chest physician, radiologist, surgeon, pathologist, oncologist, palliative care specialist and lung cancer nurse. Further investigation may be inappropriate if frail or patient does not want to pursue diagnosis/Rx. Always determine patient's performance status (see Box) before deciding on investigations (and Rx) as this can help determine the approach to management.

Several simple investigations can be carried out during the first hospital appointment of a patient with suspected lung cancer: *CXR* (if not already arranged), *spirometry* (before biopsy or surgery; may require formal lung function), *ECG* (before considering Rx), *bloods* (Na^+, Ca^{2+}, LFTs, U&E and clotting), *pleural aspiration* (↓USS if effusion), *lymph node FNA* (supraclavicular or cervical; if enlarged) and *sputum cytology* (rarely indicated).

The following can be subsequently arranged.

Radiology

- **Contrast-enhanced staging CT (chest, neck, liver, adrenals):** Determines potential sites for biopsy (including metastasis).

2.9.2 Eastern Cooperative Oncology Group (ECOG)/World Health Organisation (WHO) Performance Status (PS)

PS 0: Fully active, able to carry on all pre-disease performance without restriction.

PS 1: Restricted in physically strenuous activity but ambulatory and able to carry out work of a light or sedentary nature, e.g. light house work, office work.

PS 2: Ambulatory and capable of all self-care but unable to carry out any work activities. Up and about > 50% of waking hours.

PS 3: Capable of only limited self-care, confined to bed or chair > 50% of waking hours.

PS 4: Completely disabled. Cannot carry on any self-care. Totally confined to bed or chair.

PS 5: Dead

- **Ultrasound (neck or liver):** Identifies enlarged nodes or liver metastasis suitable for biopsy.
- **CT/MRI head:** If brain metastasis suspected (e.g. neurological signs, headache, seizure, vomiting) and sometimes performed in patients where curative Rx is planned (e.g. surgery).
- **Bone scan:** If suspected bony metastasis (e.g. pain, fracture, $\uparrow Ca^{2+}$/ALP).
- **Positron Emission Tomography (PET):** Tumours show $\uparrow$uptake of radiolabelled 18-fluorodeoxyglucose (FDG) due to $\uparrow$metabolic activity. False negatives (e.g. BAC, carcinoid; $\downarrow$metabolic activity) and false positives (e.g. infection) are possible. Considered prior to radical Rx or to assess any nodes of uncertain significance.

Histological diagnosis

Choice of biopsy largely depends on tumour location. Also ensure patient is suitable (e.g. PS, unlikely to result in harm, will influence management, adequate FEV_1, clotting checked ± reversed). Also important to consider the need for a larger specimen for molecular analysis (e.g. epidermal growth factor receptor (EGFR) activating mutations; discussed hereunder).

- **Bronchoscopy:** Generally suitable for central tumours only, NOT all! Samples obtained by endobronchial biopsy, brushing or washing. Endobronchial ultrasound (EBUS) can help obtain lymph node FNA samples ('blind transbronchial needle aspiration' (TBNA) less commonly performed nowadays). **NB:** bronchoscopy can also help with the planning of surgery (e.g. vocal cord paralysis = inoperable; tumour position < 2 cm from carina requires pneumonectomy while those confined to lobar bronchus may be resectable with lobectomy).
- **Radiology-guided biopsy:** Usually reserved for any mass NOT amenable to bronchoscopy. Performed by either CT or US. Risk of pneumothorax is high ($\approx$ 20%).
- **Surgical biopsy:** Can be achieved via mediastinoscopy/ mediastinotomy (if potential lymph node involvement), VATS or during the definitive operation itself (e.g. occasionally performed w/o preoperative histology if high index of suspicion that cancer is potentially curative).

STAGING

Lung cancers are staged according to the **TNM system** (Tables 2.7–2.9). Important when deciding on Rx, esp potential for curative surgical procedure. Although SCLC is classified according to TNM, traditionally it has been staged as *limited* (confined to ipsilateral hemithorax, including ipsilateral mediastinal and supraclavicular lymph nodes) or *extensive* (extends beyond).

TREATMENT

The followings are general Rx options for patients with NSCLC and SCLC. Rx of oncological emergencies (page 245), pleural effusion (page 210) and palliative care (page 114) are covered elsewhere.

☠ Significant life-threatening side effects can occur with lung cancer medications and they should only be prescribed by a specialist ☠.

Table 2.7 Staging of lung cancer

Primary tumour (T)

Tx	Tumour proven by presence of malignant cells in sputum or bronchial washings but not visualised by imaging or bronchoscopy.
T0	No evidence of 1° tumour.
Tis	Carcinoma *in situ* (from histology following resection).
T1	≤ 3 cm, surrounded by lung or visceral pleura, without bronchoscopic evidence of invasion more proximal than the lobar bronchus. **T1a(mi):** Minimally invasive carcinoma (pathology-proven; irrespectively of size). **T1a:** ≤ 1 cm. **T1b:** > 1 cm but ≤ 2 cm. **T1c:** > 2 cm but ≤ 3 cm.
T2	> 3 cm but ≤ 5 cm; *or* involving main bronchus (without the carina), invading visceral pleura, associated with atelectasis or obstructive pneumonitis that extends to the hilum. **T2a:** > 3 cm but ≤ 4 cm. **T2b:** > 4 cm but ≤ 5 cm.
T3	> 5 cm but ≤ 7 cm; *or* directly invades the parietal pleural, chest wall (inc superior sulcus tumours), diaphragm, phrenic nerve, mediastinal pleura, parietal pericardium; *or* in the main bronchus; *or* associated atelectasis or obstructive pneumonitis of the entire lung; *or* separate nodule(s) in the same lobe.
T4	> 7 cm; any size and invading: mediastinum, heart, great vessels, trachea, recurrent laryngeal nerve, oesophagus, vertebral body, carina or a separate nodule(s) in a different ipsilateral lobe.

Regional lymph nodes (N)

Nx	Cannot be assessed.
N0	None.
N1	Ipsilateral peribronchial and/or ipsilateral hilar lymph nodes and intrapulmonary nodes (inc involvement by direct extension).
N2	Ipsilateral mediastinal and/or subcarinal lymph node(s).
N3	Contralateral mediastinal, contralateral hilar, ipsilateral or contralateral scalene, or supraclavicular lymph node(s).

(Continued)

Table 2.7 Staging of lung cancer (*Continued*)

Primary tumour (T)

Distant metastasis (M)

Mx	Distant metastasis cannot be assessed.
M0	No distant metastasis.
M1	Distant metastasis: **M1a:** Separate nodule(s) in a contralateral lobe, pleural nodules or malignant pleural/pericardial effusion. **M1b:** Solitary extrathoracic metastasis (extrathoracic organs). **M1c:** Multiple extrathoracic metastasis (either in single or multiple organs).

Table 2.8 Staging of lung cancer

	N0	N1	N2	N3	M1a any N	M1b any N	M1c any N
T1a	IA1	IIB	IIIA	IIIB	IVA	IVA	IVB
T1b	IA2	IIB	IIIA	IIIB	IVA	IVA	IVB
T1c	IA3	IIB	IIIA	IIIB	IVA	IVA	IVB
T2a	IB	IIB	IIIA	IIIB	IVA	IVA	IVB
T2b	IIA	IIB	IIIA	IIIB	IVA	IVA	IVB
T3	IIB	IIIA	IIIB	IIIC	IVA	IVA	IVB
T4	IIIA	IIIA	IIIB	IIIC	IVA	IVA	IVB

Goldstraw P et al. J Thorac Oncol 2016; 11: 39-51.

NSCLC

Surgery: Offered as curative procedure whenever possible, i.e. a fit patient *and* potentially resectable; mostly stages I and II; rarely IIA with adjuvant chemotherapy/radiotherapy; not IIIB or IV. Fitness for surgery is often determined by a combination of global risk score (e.g. *Thoracoscore*), age, lung function (FEV$_1$, TLCO; + predicted 'post-resection' values), CV status (+ previous

Table 2.9 Survival from lung cancer at different TNM stages.
(Reference as above)

Stage	Survival with treatment at 60 months (%)
IA1	90–92
IA2	83–85
IA3	77–80
IB	68–73
IIA	60–65
IIB	53–56
IIIA	36–41
IIIB	24–26
IIIC	12–13
IVA	10
IVB	0

NB: all measurements are made in the greatest dimension.

CVA/TIA), other comorbidities, nutritional status and occasionally objective measures of exercise capacity (e.g. 6MWT or CPET). Options include *lobectomy* (or bilobectomy), *pneumonectomy*, *sleeve resection* (lobectomy + removal of a section of bronchus) or more 'lung-preserving' surgery, i.e. *segmentectomy* or *wedge-resection*. **Adjuvant chemotherapy** is chemotherapy (a cisplatin-based combination) following a complete surgical resection. It can ↑survival and is considered by oncologist in patients with NSCLC. **Neo-adjuvant chemotherapy** (pre-operative) is occasionally offered to 'down-stage' a tumour. Postoperatively, patients are followed up every 6–12 months for ≈ 5 yrs with a CXR ± CT to ensure no recurrence. If histology reveals that the resection margins were NOT clear then postoperative chemotherapy/radiotherapy offered.
Chemotherapy: Offered to stage III or IV with good PS (0, 1, occasionally 2; ↑toxicity with ↓PS). Generally limited survival gains but ↑Sx control/QoL. Optimum is **combination chemotherapy** (> 1 drug). First-line regimens use several cycles of a combination of drugs, often gemcitabine (or docetaxel, paclitaxel, vinorelbine) *plus*

a platinum drug (carboplatin or cisplatin). Monotherapy is offered if unable to tolerate combination. Patients are monitored using CT (usually after two cycles) to determine whether the response is: complete (disappearance) or partial (> 30% reduction), versus progressive (> 20% increase) or stable (no change, < 30% reduction or < 20% increase) disease.

Other agents: EGFR inhibitors can be used to Rx patients with proven activating mutations of EGFR (small proportion of NSCLC; typically never-smoking females ± Asians): erlotinib 150 mg po od (TARCEVA) or gefitinib 250 mg po od (IRESSA). NSCLC associated with an anaplastic lymphoma kinase fusion gene can be Rx with an oral tyrosine kinase inhibitor: crizotinib 250 mg po od (XALKORI), ceritinib 450 mg po od (ZYKADIA), alectinib 600 mg po od (ALECENSA) or brigatinib 90 mg po od increased to 180 mg po od after 7 days (ALUNBRIG). Pembrolizumab (KEYTRUDA) is mAb that binds to the programmed death-1 receptor to potentiate an immune response to tumour cells. It is a first- or second-line option for locally advanced or metastatic PD-L1-positive NSCLC if the tumour expresses PD-L1 (≥ 50% tumour proportion score)[NICE]. It is administered ivi (200 mg every 3 wks). Atezolizumab (TECENTRIQ) and nivolumab (OPDIVO Opdivo) are similar mAb and alternatives.

Radiotherapy: Can be radical (curative-intent; high dose), used to control disease (high dose) or for Sx relief (low dose). *Radical radiotherapy* is offered to stages I–III NSCLC with PS 0-1, who are resectable (discussed earlier) but are medically <u>un</u>fit or have declined surgery. Always perform lung function beforehand. Continuous hyperfractionated accelerated radiotherapy (CHART) is often used: small radiation doses (e.g. 54 Gy) tds for 12 days. Stereotactic ablative radiotherapy (SABR)/stereotactive body radiation (SBRT) can deliver high-radiation doses to small early stage cancers. *Palliative radiotherapy* can be given to patients with no metastatic disease + good PS (able to tolerate a high-dose regimen) to modestly ↑survival. *Low-dose radiotherapy* is used to relieve Sx (e.g. pain).

Radiofrequency ablation (RFA): Probe inserted under CT-guidance into a tumour or nodule to ablate the tissue using heat generated from a high-frequency alternating current. Used for early stage disease (size < 5 cm) in patients unsuitable for surgery/radiotherapy.

SCLC
Vital to be assessed for Rx promptly (< 1 wk of diagnosis).
Surgery: May be appropriate with limited stage SCLC (if T1-2a N0 M0) BUT this is very rare (disease usually extensive at presentation). Preoperative brain imaging, bone scans and PET are usually requested to be certain metastases are excluded, and adjuvant chemotherapy is usually given.
Concurrent chemotherapy + radiotherapy: Patients with limited stage SCLC should receive combination chemotherapy, usually etoposide + cisplatin (or carboplatin if ↓PS, comorbidity, ↑U&E) and be considered for concurrent (during first or second cycle) consolidation radiotherapy (only if PS 0/1 and disease encompassed in a radical radiotherapy volume). Alternatively give radiotherapy within 6 wks of chemotherapy completion if unfit for concurrent Rx but responded to chemotherapy. Prophylactic cranial radiotherapy is also given to those with limited disease. *Patients with extensive SCLC* receive chemotherapy (ONLY if suitable) before palliative thoracic radiotherapy (ONLY if response to chemotherapy).

OTHER IMPORTANT TUMOURS
Mesothelioma
Malignant tumour of the mesothelium; most often the pleura but also peritoneum, pericardium or tunica vaginalis (testes). Usually the result of asbestos exposure (see Box); ≈ 90% of cases have documented exposure (not always ↑dose). Other rare causes: erionite fibres (Turkey), Simian virus 40, ionizing radiation, chest injury, genetic predisposition (BAP1 gene) or 'spontaneous'. Typically presents with pleural effusion (usually unilateral; investigation page 210), thick pleural rind, chest pain and constitutional Sx (e.g. ↓Wt, sweating).

Investigations
Pleural fluid aspiration: Exudate, often blood-stained (cytology frequently positive). ☠ Avoid repeated aspiration as tumour may track ☠.

Radiology: CT may reveal an effusion with pleural thickening, nodularity, contrast-enhancement ± lung encasement (loss of volume). The *mediastinal pleura* is usually involved. May have local invasion (ribs, chest wall, diaphragm, upper abdomen, mediastinal structures, heart or contralateral thorax). If diagnostic doubt, PET may distinguish benign/malignant pleural disease.
Biopsy: Usually US/CT guided or occasionally by VATs (+ talc pleurodesis). Broadly, *epithelioid* (similar to adenocarcinoma; better prognosis), *sarcomatoid* or *mixed* (biphasic) histology.

Treatment

Poor survival rates (median 4–12 months). Adequate analgesia and palliative measures are vital and should be started early (page 114).

2.9.3 Asbestos-related lung disease

Naturally occurring fibre. Can be curly (serpentine; e.g. chrysotile, white) or straight (amphibole; e.g. crocidolite, blue → most carcinogenic). Exposure usually occupational. Typically a long latency from exposure by inhalation until disease, ≈ 30 years. Encourage patients with disease and known asbestos exposure (not plaques) to seek compensation from government and employer (civil law). Notify all asbestos-related deaths to coroner. Several different asbestos-related processes can occur:

Benign pleural plaques: Usually asymptomatic (unless extensive) and NOT pre-malignant.
Benign pleural effusions: Usually small, unilateral and asymptomatic.
Benign diffuse pleural thickening: Symptomatic extensive fibrosis (decortication can be tried).
Benign rounded atelectasis ('folded lung'): Contracting fibrotic pleura twists and traps portion of lung (classical 'comet tail' appearance on CT), rarely Sx or require Rx.
Asbestosis: Fibrotic process (no Rx; supportive care only).
Mesothelioma
Lung cancer

Chest wall neuropathic pain may require atypical analgesia (e.g. amitriptyline, pregabalin, gabapentin), nerve block or palliative radiotherapy. Manage pleural effusions with a drain ± talc pleurodesis (**NB:** lung may not re-expand, i.e. 'trapped lung'), VATs or long-term indwelling drain (page 222). Chemotherapy is reserved for patients with a good PS, usually pemetrexed + cisplatin (carboplatin if ↑risk of toxicity).

Carcinoid tumours
Uncommon 1° neuroendocrine lung tumour. Usually slow-growing and benign; aggressive subtypes with metastatic potential are rare. Classically an isolated endobronchial tumour → wheeze/stridor, haemoptysis, persistent collapse/consolidation. ≈ 1% have carcinoid syndrome (flushing, ↑HR/↓BP, sweats and diarrhoea). CXR/CT will reveal an isolated and well-defined tumour. Usually accessible by bronchoscopy (endobronchial) and appear as cherry red (vascular), well-demarcated and covered in intact epithelium. Brushings often adequate for diagnosis (risk of significant bleeding with biopsy; clinical diagnosis often accepted!). Rx for isolated pulmonary carcinoid is surgery or occasionally endobronchial resection. Carcinoid syndrome requires serotonin antagonists (e.g. octreotide 50–200 mcg sc od/bd/tds) but resolves after resection. Metastatic/aggressive carcinoid requires chemotherapy (optimum regimen unknown).

PULMONARY NODULES
Focal area of ↑opacification, < 3 cm in diameter. Most are incidental and benign (granuloma, adenoma or hamartoma), but some represent an early 1° malignancy (≈ 1–2% in smokers) or metastasis. Several characteristics suggest ↑malignancy risk: ↑age, smoking, known extrathoracic malignancy, > 1 cm, ↑size over time (may be slow growing), contrast enhancement (> 15 Hounsfield units), FDG uptake on PET, irregular/spiculated margin, associated ground-glass or thick-walled cavitation.

Management

Discuss each individual case in MDT meeting. Options include radiological surveillance for small incidental nodules < 8 mm (usually over 12–24 months), biopsy (if > 8 mm), PET (**NB:** false negatives and positives are possible), surgery (e.g. wedge resection or segmentectomy; if nodule increases in size, patient is ↑risk or PET is FDG avid) or occasionally radiotherapy (proven malignancy but surgery inappropriate). Important guidelines and a risk of malignancy calculator are available from the BTS:

- https://www.brit-thoracic.org.uk/guidelines-and-quality-standards/pulmonary-nodules/
- https://www.brit-thoracic.org.uk/guidelines-and-quality-standards/pulmonary-nodules/bts-pulmonary-nodule-risk-prediction-calculator/

Tip: Cancer Research UK and BTS have also produced a free app for iPhone and Android, which includes the risk calculators and summary information from the above guidelines (Pulmonary Nodule Risk).

LUNG TRANSPLANTATION

An option for many chronic and progressive end-stage respiratory conditions inc COPD, IPF, CF, α1-antitrypsin deficiency, IPAH, other ILD, bronchiectasis and PHT (order of frequency). Deciding whether transplantation is appropriate depends on several factors and is determined by the UK transplant centre (Harefield, Papworth, Birmingham, Manchester & Newcastle). Deciding whether to refer (and the timing of this referral) can be very difficult and should be consultant-led (Box 2.10.1). If referring, complete the universal **'UK Adult Lung and Heart-Lung Transplantation Referral Proforma'** (available on all transplant centre websites).

Transplants can be single lung, bilateral, heart-lung or living lobar transplantation (lower lobes grafted from two suitable living adult donors; rare in the UK). Survival rates post-transplant are ≈ 85% at 1 yr, ≈ 60% at 3 yrs and ≈ 50% at 5 yrs. Chance of death is highest in first year (infection or graft failure most common). ☠ Be alert

2.10.1 Suggested referral criteria for lung transplantation

The following criteria are NOT absolute and serve as a guide only. If in doubt consult transplant centre. High waiting list mortalities suggest that referrals are often made too late!

Refer for progressive, chronic, end-stage lung disease *despite optimal medical therapy* **plus**:

- Age < 65 yrs
- Life-expectancy ≈ 2–3 yrs (or less, but note that mean time on waiting list > 12 months)
- Patient wishes to be considered
- Still able to walk (despite being functionally impaired)
- No significant renal, cardiac or liver comorbidity
- BMI > 17 but < 30
- No recent history of malignancy (< 2 yrs) or substantial likelihood of recurrence
- Incurable chronic infection (inc. HIV, Hepatitis B and C)
- Absence of factors that might impact outcome, rehabilitation or recovery (e.g. Ψ disorder, lack of social network or consistent lack of compliance)

As a general rule the following are performed prior to referral: Full lung function, 6MWT, sputum MC&S, ECG, Echo (± stress echo/angiogram), HRCT, routine bloods, viral serology (HIV, CMV, HCV, HBV).

to possible complications (below), esp any ustained ↓spirometric values (> 10%) ☠. Liaise with transplant centre early if any complications are suspected! See Box.

MMUNOSUPPRESSIVE AGENTS

.egimens are initiated by transplant centres and must be continued .ifelong. Usually a combination of **tacrolimus** or **ciclosporin**, **mycophenolate mofetil (MMF)** or **azathioprine** and **prednisolone** (Box 2.10.3):

Tacrolimus: Macrolide and calcineurin inhibitor (avoid if macrolide allergy). Available as intermediate-release (bd po)

(ADOPORT, PROGRAF, CAPXION, TACNI, VIVADEX and MODIGRAF) and prolonged-release preparations (od po) (ADVAGRAF). Closely monitor for nephrotoxicity, ↑BP, neurotoxicity and glucose intolerance (common). *Some notable drug interactions* inc antibiotics (aminoglycosides, macrolides), ACEI, CCBs, diuretics (potassium-sparing and aldosterone antagonists) and NSAIDs.

2.10.2 Transplant complications

Early graft dysfunction: First few days postoperative. Pulmonary infiltrates and ↓PO$_2$. Related to lung ischaemia/reperfusion. Very high mortality. Rx is supportive (usually in ITU).

Acute rejection: Very common in first 3 months (rare > 1 yr). Onset can be insidious with non-specific findings. Suspect with ↓spirometry (>10%). Always refer back to transplant centre. Transbronchial biopsy shows perivascular lymphocytic infiltrates. Rx = pulsed IV methylprednisolone.

Chronic rejection: Affects ≈ 50% of patients at 5 yrs (rare < 6 months). Immune-mediated but often other triggers (e.g. infection inc. CMV, or GORD). Suspect with insidious onset of SOB ± progressive airflow obstruction (↓FEV$_1$/FEF). Transbronchial biopsy shows bronchiolitis obliterans (low yield). Rx any triggers and seek advice on changes or additions to immunosuppression. Prognosis very poor. Re-transplantation is controversial.

Surgical: Anastomotic stenosis or dehiscence may require repeat intervention (seek advice).

Infection: Bacterial (esp *PSEUDOMONAS*), CMV (esp seropositive donor to seronegative recipient) and aspergillus infection are all common.

Malignancy: Particularly lymphoma.

Recurrence of primary lung disease

Drug-related complication (see below)

2.10.3 Important points

- Always consult BNF when co-prescribing (many different drug interactions)
- Multiple SEs and risk of toxicity
- Never alter dosages without consulting specialist
- Always prescribe *tacrolimus* and *ciclosporin* by *brand name only* and never switch brands unless specialist advice and only with careful supervision and therapeutic monitoring (risk of toxicity or rejection)
- Therapeutic monitoring is available (esp. if toxicity or rejection suspected)

Ciclosporin: Calcineurin inhibitor (CAPIMUNE, CAPSORIN, DEXIMUNE, NEORAL, SANDIMMUN). 💀Markedly nephrotoxic 💀. *Some notable drug interactions* inc antibiotics (aminoglycosides, macrolides, quinolones, trimethoprim, vancomycin), ACEI, allopurinol, amiodarone, anti-epileptics (carbamazepine, phenytoin), diuretics (thiazides, potassium-sparing and aldosterone antagonists), statins, CCBs and tacrolimus.

Mycophenolate Mofetil (CELLCEPT): Metabolised to active mycophenolic acid (inhibitor of purine synthesis). Risk of bone marrow suppression. Warn patients of signs (e.g. bleeding, bruising or infection) and monitor FBC regularly. Less potential for drug interactions (**NB:** rifampicin can ↓plasma concentration).

Azathioprine (IMURAN): Purine analogue. Metabolised by thiopurine methyltransferase (TPMT) → always check TPMT test before commencing (page 185). Risk of bone marrow suppression. Warn patients of signs (e.g. bleeding, bruising or infection) and monitor FBC regularly. Beware co-prescription with trimethoprim or allopurinol (↑toxicity).

PALIATIVE CARE AND SUBCUTANEOUS PUMPS

Important points:

- Palliative care is not only an important aspect of Rx for pulmonary malignancy but also many 'end-stage' non-malignant respiratory conditions (e.g. COPD, CF, ILD Box 2.11.1).
- Under-prescribed due to stigma of being a 'final measure': ensure good communication with patient, relatives and nurses as to reasons for use.
- Palliative care, Macmillan and hospital pain teams will help if unsure of the indications or how to set up SC pumps.

2.11.1 Some potential pitfalls

Missing ↑Ca^{2+} as the cause of confusion/agitation, constipation and/or pain.

Missing other potentially reversible/easily treatable conditions that can worsen symptoms in terminal illness (e.g. ↓Hb, pleural effusion, PE, SVCO, cord compression).

Forgetting to prescribe regular simple analgesia (e.g. paracetamol), which could otherwise ↓ opiate requirement (and ADRs).

Forgetting that palliative radiotherapy can be used to manage pain (e.g. bony pain).

COMMON SYMPTOMS
Pain

Start with simple analgesia and ↑according to WHO analgesic ladder: broadly non-opioids (paracetamol or NSAIDs) → weak opioids (codeine or tramadol) → strong opioids (morphine, diamorphine or fentanyl). ALWAYS ensure adequate PRN analgesia is also prescribed for breakthrough pain. ☠ Take care with renal failure (opioids or NSAIDs) and when converting doses between opioids or switching modes of administration (sc/iv/po) → consult BNF ☠.

Morphine is usually required for patients with pain relating to lung cancer (regular dose + breakthrough dose):

1. *Regular analgesia* = 40–60 mg morphine/24 h (divided 4-hourly if immediate-release, or bd if MR preparation). Start with immediate-release and convert to MR once pain is well controlled.
2. *Breakthrough analgesia* = 1/6th of regular morphine dose as immediate-release morphine PRN/4-hourly. Typically start with 5–10 mg.

Always monitor and Rx any SEs (e.g. prophylactic laxatives and antiemetics). If possible, continue regular simple analgesia (paracetamol or NSAIDs). Give opiates a chance to work; assess regularly and ↑ dose of regular analgesia if breakthrough analgesia is being used frequently. ALWAYS consider alternatives, e.g. steroids for liver capsule pain or radiotherapy/IV pamidronate 90 mg for localised bony pain.

Dyspnoea

ALWAYS ensure optimum medical Rx of any underlying condition (e.g. bronchodilators for COPD). Also consider any coexisting pathology. This is very common with pulmonary malignancy and Rx can alleviate aggravated SOB, e.g. anaemia (→blood transfusion), pleural effusion (→drainage), PE (→LMWH), pneumonia (→antibiotics), lymphangitis carcinomatosis (→steroids) or upper airway obstruction (→debulking ± stenting).

Managing dyspnoea

Mainstay of Rx is opiates, e.g. morphine sulphate 2.5–5 mg po/4 h (ORAMORPH) but monitor for signs of respiratory suppression! Consider use of O_2, especially with demonstrable hypoxia (often short-burst oxygen therapy [SBOT]) but remember this may restrict activities/generate psychological dependence. Non-pharmacological options include reassurance (↑SOB with anxiety or hyperventilation), avoiding claustrophobic situations, encouraging to sit upright (↑chest expansion) and fan blowing.

Cough

Rx underlying cause. Try codeine linctus ± methadone linctus
(↑ duration of action). Many will require opiates: codeine
phosphate 30 mg po qds often sufficient but may require morphine
sulphate 2.5–5 mg po/4 h (ORAMORPH). Neb local anaesthetic
an option (e.g. 5 mL 0.25% bupivacaine tds): avoid in asthmatics
(bronchoconstriction); NB risk of aspiration.

Anxiety

Often (but not always) linked to SOB. Mainstay of Rx is short-
term use of benzodiazepines e.g. lorazepam 0.5–1 mg po or
diazepam 2–5 mg po. ☠ ALWAYS beware respiratory suppression
☠. Consider longer-term amitriptyline (75–150 mg po on) or
citalopram (20–40 mg po od), particularly for any depression
associated with non-malignant conditions.

Nausea, vomiting and anorexia

N&V are very common with advanced cancer (tumour- and
Rx-related, e.g. opiates or chemotherapy). Where possible,
identify cause before starting Rx. Some initial options include
metoclopramide 10 mg tds po/iv/im (prokinetic), haloperidol 1.5 mg
bd po (metabolic causes), cyclizine 50 mg tds po/iv/im (↑ ICP) or
ondansetron 8–24 mg po, 1–2 h before emetogenic chemotherapy.
Also see SC syringe divers given hereunder. Anorexia is common
and can be improved short term with dexamethasone 2–4 mg bd po.

CONTINUOUS SUBCUTANEOUS INFUSIONS

Parental route often required, especially with N&V or an inability to
take po medications. Continuous SC pumps give smooth symptom
control, esp for pain, but are also useful for other Sx, e.g. nausea, xs
secretions, agitation. They avoid cannulation and only require a single
24-h prescription (no delays in drug administration on busy wards).
  Contents of subcutaneous pump (Box 2.11.2):

1. **Diamorphine (or morphine sulphate):** Calculate dose needed for
   24 h prescription from the past 24 h's requirements (if variable,
   look at longer-term trend). For breakthrough pain ensure a

subcutaneous dose (preferable; intermittent bolus is kindest) equivalent to 1/10th to 1/6th of total 24-hour subcutaneous infusion dose. If taking other opioids (or routes), use the following rough guide to calculate conversions:

$$1 \text{ mg diamorphine sc/im} = 1.5 \text{ mg morphine sc/im}$$
$$= 3 \text{ mg morphine po}$$
$$= 15 \text{ mg tramadol po}$$
$$= 35 \text{ mg codeine po/im}$$

(For conversion from fentanyl, see its entry in main drugs section). **NB:** these equivalent doses only apply for specific route(s) of each drug stated, as bioavailability can vary widely with routes. Also, it does not take into account duration of action, although this can be ignored if 24 h requirements for each drug are calculated. At high-opioid doses, conversion factors become less reliable – err on the conservative side and gradually titrate up.

2. **Antiemetic:** Choose from (generally start at lowest dose):
   - Metoclopramide 30–100 mg/24 h: (esp for pro-motility fx slow gastric emptying; but CI if GI obstruction with abdominal pain!).
   - Haloperidol 0.5–5 mg/24 h: good general antiemetic.
   - Cyclizine 50 mg tds sc/po/24 h: good if cause unknown or multifactorial.
   - Levomepromazine 5–12.5 mg/24 h: good if cause unknown or multifactorial (↑doses to 25–50 mg/h if sedation needed and patient not ambulant).

3. **Optional extras**
   - Drugs to ↓respiratory secretions:
     - Glycopyrronium 0.6–1.2 mg/24 h.
     - Hyoscine hydrobromide 0.6–2.4 mg/24 h: normally sedative but can → paradoxical agitation. ↑risk of seizures.
   - Sedatives, e.g. midazolam 10–60 mg/24 h if restlessness or agitation is the solitary symptom. Consider levomepromazine if not responsive to midazolam. Care/↓dose if elderly, respiratory depression, benzodiazepine-naive.

Table 2.10 Compatibility^a of specific three-drug combinations: diamorphine and antiemetic and one other 'optional extra' drug

Diamorphine *plus*	Glycopyrronium	Hyoscine hydrobromide	Midazolam
Metoclopramide	Not recommended	Not recommended	Compatible^a
Haloperidol	Compatible^a	Compatible^a	Compatible^a
Levomepromazine	Compatible^a	Compatible^a	Compatible^a

^a Compatibility is restricted to usual dose ranges of the drugs.

2.11.2 Compatibility of drugs in syringe drivers

It is advised that only 2 or 3 drugs are used per syringe driver. All antiemetics listed above are compatible with diamorphine and morphine. For addition of 'optional extras', see Table 2.10; for all other combinations, check with the hospital pharmacy or drug information office. Out-of-hours authoritative information on compatibility (and other palliative care prescribing issues) can be found at the excellent website www.palliativedrugs.com.

Example prescription

Prescribe each drug individually in the 'regular prescriptions' section of the drug chart, as shown in Figure 2.6.

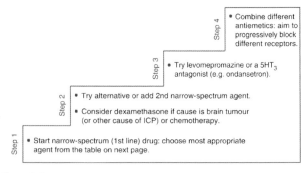

Step 4
- Combine different antiemetics: aim to progressively block different receptors.

Step 3
- Try levomepromazine or a 5HT$_3$ antagonist (e.g. ondansetron).

Step 2
- Try alternative or add 2nd narrow-spectrum agent.
- Consider dexamethasone if cause is brain tumour (or other cause of ICP) or chemotherapy.

Step 1
- Start narrow-spectrum (1st line) drug: choose most appropriate agent from the table on next page.

Figure 2.6

GENERAL POINTERS IN CHRONIC PAIN/PALLIATIVE CARE

Laxatives: Give with opiates as Px rather than later as Rx.

Simple analgesia: Do not forget as often effective, e.g. regular paracetamol.

Breakthrough analgesia: Always write up in case regular medications become insufficient (Box 2.11.3). Oral opiates such as morphine sulphate immediate release solution (e.g. ORAMORPH) often best; 1/6 of regular 24-h opiate equivalent dose is usually sufficient (discussed earlier). If ↓GCS or ↓swallow add sc or iv drugs (e.g. morphine).

2.11.3 Graseby syringe drivers: mm (instead of mL) per unit time

This type of syringe driver is common in the UK (esp. in specialist palliative care settings). Infusions are given in millimetres (mm) rather than millilitres (mL) per unit time. There are two types: for each unit on the 'rate' dial, the MS16 (blue) delivers 2 mm/h, but the MS26 (green) delivers 48 mm/day. Examples of prescriptions of a syringe to be given over 24 h:

MS16: 'Diamorphine 60 mg over 24 h as subcutaneous infusion via syringe driver. Mix with water for injection to a length of 48 mm in syringe, set at rate of 2 mm/h'

MS26: 'Diamorphine 60 mg over 24 h as subcutaneous infusion via syringe driver. Mix with water for injection to a length of 48 mm in syringe, set at rate of 48 mm/24 h'

☠ Confusing mm with mL or confusing the two types of driver can lead to significant differences in rate of drug delivery ☠.

Fentanyl patches: Smooth pain control w/o multiple injections or tablets (just change patch every 3rd day). Also less constipating. ☠ Only use if stable opioid requirements; long action means dose overestimation can be fatal ☠.

Steroids: Consider for nausea, as pain adjuvant (esp liver capsule pain), and for short-term Rx of ↓appetite: Get specialist help.
Always consider new causes of pain/distress: esp if patient unable to give Hx: often treatable, iatrogenic or can be disguised/made worse by more analgesia, e.g. opiate-induced constipation, patient positioning, UTI, urinary retention, mental anguish (esp 'unfinished business'), pathological fractures.

PULMONARY HYPERTENSION

Many different causes (Table 2.11). Pulmonary hypertension (PHT) is defined as a **resting mean PAP (mPAP) $\geq$ 25 to 20 mmHg** at right-heart catheter (normal mPAP $\approx$ 8–20 mmHg). Pulmonary capillary wedge pressure (PCWP) usually normal ($\leq$ 15 mmHg), except when PHT arises from left heart disease or is multifactorial (Groups 2 and 5; below). ☠ **Vital:** do NOT confuse mPAP at right heart catheter with the echo reading of systolic PAP (sPAP); although sPAP > 40 mmHg usually implies an mPAP > 25 mmHg ☠.

Underlying pathophysiology is vasoconstriction, vessel wall remodelling/hypertrophy, fibrotic changes and thrombosis. Imbalances between vasodilators/vasoconstrictors, platelet activating/inhibiting factors and regulators of vascular tone have all been implicated. Ultimately → ↑pulmonary vascular resistance → right ventricular failure. *Sxs and signs* relate to RV dysfunction, e.g. SOB on exertion (see Box), peripheral oedema, RV heave, ↑JVP or splitting of S2 with loud P2. There may also be signs of the underlying causes, e.g. scleroderma, clubbing.

NATIONAL PULMONARY HYPERTENSION SERVICE

Established in the UK and Ireland to help coordinate the diagnosis, offer prognosis, make complex management decisions (involving expensive pharmacotherapy), review progress and gather data for

Table 2.11 Clinical classification of pulmonary hypertension

1. Pulmonary arterial hypertension

1.1	Idiopathic (IPAH)		Incidence 1/million (F>M); mean age 36
1.2	Heritable (HPAH)	1.2.1 Bone morphogenetic protein receptor type 2 (BMPR2)	Heritable ≈ 10% of IPAH cases. BMPR2 (most common) and ALK1 are part of the TGF-β receptor superfamily.
		1.2.2 Other mutations (e.g. Activin receptor-like kinase 1 gene (ALK1), endoglin (with or without haemorrhagic telangiectasia))	
1.3	Drug- and toxin-induced		Careful Hx (many drugs/toxins).
1.4	Associated with (APAH)	1.4.1 Connective tissue diseases	APAH ≈ 50% of patients. Consider systemic sclerosis, RA, SLE. Sjögren's & dermatomyositis. Common in
		1.4.2 HIV infection	HIV (0.5%), portal hypertension (≈ 5%)
		1.4.3 Portal hypertension	and with L-R shunts.
		1.4.4 Congenital heart disease	
		1.4.5 Schistosomiasis	
1'	Pulmonary veno-occlusive disease and/or pulmonary capillary haemangiomatosis	1'.1 Idiopathic	Hard to classify. HRCT features ± biopsy.

(Continued)

Table 2.11 Clinical classification of pulmonary hypertension (*Continued*)

	1'.2 Heritable	
	1'.2.1 Eukaryotic translation initiation factor 2-α kinase 4 (ELF2AK4) mutation	
	1'.2.2 Other mutations	
	1'.3 Drugs, toxins and radiation-induced	
	1'.4 Associated with:	
	1'.4.1 Connective tissue disease	
	1'.4.2 HIV infection	
2. Pulmonary hypertension due to left heart disease		
2.1	LV systolic dysfunction	↑Pulmonary capillary wedge pressure.
2.2	LV diastolic dysfunction	
2.3	Valvular disease	
2.4	Congenital/acquired left heart inflow/outflow tract obstruction and congenital cardiomyopathies	
2.5	Congenital/acquired pulmonary veins stenosis	

(Continued)

Table 2.11 Clinical classification of pulmonary hypertension (*Continued*)

3. Pulmonary hypertension due to lung diseases and/or hypoxia

3.1	COPD		Commonest in clinical practise and result of chronic hypoxia. PHT confers additional morbidity and ↓prognosis. Consider referral to specialist centre for 'PHT (Sx) out of proportion to the underlying lung disease' (esp > 40 mmHg).
3.2	ILD		
3.3	Other pulmonary diseases with mixed restrictive and obstructive pattern		
3.4	Sleep-disordered breathing		
3.5	Alveolar hypoventilation disorders		
3.6	Chronic exposure to high altitude		
3.7	Developmental abnormalities		
4. Chronic thromboembolic pulmonary hypertension (CTEPH)			
4.1	Chronic thromboembolic pulmonary hypertension		Organised clot + vascular remodelling.
4.2	Other pulmonary artery obstructions	4.2.1 Angiosarcoma	
		4.2.2 Other intravascular tumours	
		4.2.3 Arteritis	
		4.2.4 Congenital pulmonary arteries stenoses	
		4.2.5 Parasites (hydatidosis)	

(Continued)

Table 2.11 Clinical classification of pulmonary hypertension (*Continued*)

	5. Pulmonary hypertension with unclear and/or multifactorial mechanisms	
5.1	Haematological disorders: chronic haemolytic anaemia, myeloproliferative, splenectomy	Heterogenous group of different pathologies.
5.2	Systemic disorders: sarcoidosis, pulmonary histiocytosis, lymphangioleiomyomatosis	
5.3	Metabolic disorders: glycogen storage disease, Gaucher's disease, thyroid disorders	
5.4	Others: pulmonary tumoral thrombothic microangiopathy, fibrosing mediastinitis, chronic renal failure (±dialysis), segmental pulmonary hypertension	

Source: Adapted from Eur Heart J (August 2015).

> **2.12.1 WHO functional assessment classification for PAH (modified from NYHA classification)**
>
> **Class I**   PAH w/o resulting limitation of physical activity.
> **Class II** PAH resulting in slight limitation of physical activity. Comfortable at rest. Ordinary physical activity does not cause undue SOB or fatigue, chest pain or near syncope.
> **Class III** PAH resulting in marked limitation of physical activity. Comfortable at rest. Less than ordinary physical activity causes undue SOB or fatigue, chest pain or near syncope.
> **Class IV** PAH with an inability to carry out any physical activity w/o Sxs. These patients manifest signs of right heart failure. SOB and/or fatigue may even be present at rest. Discomfort is increased by any physical activity.

research/audit. A confirmed diagnosis (i.e. right heart catheter) is NOT required prior to referral one of the specialist centres:

- **London**   Hammersmith Hospital (general)
  - Royal Brompton Hospital (adult congenital heart disease)
  - Royal Free Hospital (connective tissue disease)
  - Great Ormond Street Hospital for Children (children)
- **Cambridge**   Papworth Hospital
- **Sheffield**   Royal Hallamshire Hospital
- **Newcastle**   Freeman Hospital
- **Glasgow**   Golden Jubilee National Hospital
- **Dublin**   Mater Misericordiae University Hospital

INVESTIGATIONS FOR PHT

Aim is to make the diagnosis (**right heart catheter is gold standard!**) *and* identify any underlying cause (selective tests). **Important:** most patients ($\approx$ 90%) will have an abnormal CXR and/or ECG.

- **Right heart catheter:** Performed by specialist centre $\rightarrow$ mPAP, PCWP, cardiac output, left-to-right cardiac shunt and vasodilator responsiveness to inh NO or iv epoprostenol/adenosine (defined as $\downarrow$ mPAP > 10 (or 20%) to an mPAP < 40 mmHg with $\leftrightarrow$/$\uparrow$ cardiac output; usually < 10% patients).

- **CXR:** Cardiomegaly + $\uparrow$pulmonary arteries with pruning of peripheral vessels.
- **ECG:** Right atrial enlargement (P pulmonale inferior leads or V2), RAD and RV strain/RVH.
- **Echocardiogram:** NOT diagnostic but a useful 'screening' tool. $\uparrow$right heart chamber size with paradoxical movement of interventricular septum + TR $\pm$ pericardial effusion. sPAP can be estimated from the peak velocity of TR jet and the right atrial pressure from the IVC. Suggestive echo findings should be followed up with a right heart catheter (if appropriate).
- **Lung function:** $\downarrow$TLCO $\pm$ any evidence of underlying lung disease.
- **ABG:** $\downarrow$PO$_2$ ($\pm$ desaturation on exercise).
- **Lung and cardiac imaging:** HRCT and V/Q (or CTPA/ VQ SPECT) to rule out underlying lung disease and chronic thromboembolic disease, respectively (**NB:** V/Q more sensitive than CTPA; pulmonary angiography rarely required). Cardiac MRI can be used evaluate the RV size, morphology and function.
- **Liver USS:** If liver cirrhosis or portal hypertension suspected.
- **Blood tests:** Helpful in identifying any cause of PAH, inc LFT, HIV, TSH, ACE, autoantibodies, BNP and thrombophilia (if chronic thromboembolism).

TREATMENT

☠ **Important:** Pharmacotherapy for PAH (Group 1) should only be started by a specialist centre (<u>never</u> by non-specialists) ☠. The following serves as a guide only! The initiation of Rx depends on the vasodilator response at right heart catheter.

'Vasodilator-responders': *Calcium channel blockers* are considered first line, e.g. high-dose *nifedipine* (120–240 mg po daily) or *diltiazem* (240–720 mg po daily); relative $\downarrow$HR favours nifedipine and $\uparrow$HR favours diltiazem. Started and titrated as an inpatient with close monitoring. Only continued if a sustained response demonstrated at repeat right heart catheter. Inadequate response → additional PAH Rx started.

1. **'Non-responders':** *First-line therapy* is usually with an oral agent, typically a **phosphodiesterase type-5 inhibitor (PDE5I)** (work by ↑NO-mediated vasodilatation), e.g. sildenafil (5–20 mg po tds) or tadalafil (40 mg po od) *or* with an **endothelin receptor antagonist (ERA)**, e.g. bosentan (62.5–125 mg po bd), ambrisentan (5–10 mg po od) or macitentan (10 mg po od). Those who fail to respond/sub-optimally respond/do not tolerate Rx/deteriorate are considered for the alternative oral agent *or* trialled on dual oral therapy. Some patients are commenced on combination oral Rx from the start (e.g. ambrisentan + tadalafil). **Prostacylin analogues** are usually reserved for resistant or more severe cases (e.g. epoprostenol, treprostinil, iloprost). They have a short half-life and are most commonly administered by continuous ivi/sc infusion or by neb for iloprost. Also available is prostacyclin receptor agonist selexipag, which is indicated for long-term PAH management in patients with WHO functional classes II–III, either as combination therapy in patients insufficiently controlled with ERA and/or PDE5I or as monotherapy in patients who are not candidates for these therapies. ☠ Multiple drug interactions, risk of infection and pump failure may be life-threatening ☠.

2. **Surgical management:** Selected patients may benefit from an atrial septostomy (palliative procedure that creates a right-to-left shunt), pulmonary thromboendarterectomy (Rx of choice for proximal CTEPH) or transplantation.

Other important considerations: R/L, anticoagulation with warfarin (↑risk of VTE), domiciliary O_2, (prevent further pulmonary vasoconstriction), diuretics (for oedema), digoxin (↑cardiac output), immunisation and contraception (pregnancy is high risk and should be avoided). The median survival of NHYA class IV ≈ 6 months → consider early palliative care involvement.

PULMONARY VASCULITIS

Vasculitis is inflammation and necrosis of the *small*, *medium* or *large* blood vessels. The pulmonary vessels can be affected as part of a multi-system process (usually small vessel, i.e. arterioles/capillaries/venules). Clinical features are mainly non-specific and mimic other diseases (e.g. lung cancer), but suspect if fail to improve on initial Rx, alveolar haemorrhage (haemoptysis/significant hypoxia/↑KCO), sinus or nasal disease, associated RF/haematuria/proteinuria (dipstick) or ↑ANCA (see Box).

> ### 2.13.1 Anti-neutrophil cytoplasmic antibody (ANCA)
>
> Group of autoAbs that target Ag in the NΦ cytoplasm, either myeloperoxidase (anti-MPO) or proteinase 3 (anti-PR3). Immunofluorescence detects ANCA and differentiates between two patterns:
>
> **Perinuclear (pANCA)** → anti-MPO
> **Cytoplasmic (cANCA)** → anti-PR3
>
> If immunofluorescence is positive, an ANCA titre is to be performed; testing serum dilutions (1:4, 1:8, 1:16, 1:32 etc.) for the presence of autoAb. For example, a titre of 1:64 indicates autoAb presence in a 64-fold dilution. The higher the titre, the more ANCA is present.

INVESTIGATING VASCULITIS

Consider the following tests in the work-up of suspected pulmonary vasculitis.

CXR: Signs often non-specific and misdiagnosed (e.g. consolidation, infiltrates, effusion, bronchiectasis). May see flitting pulmonary nodules (± cavities; GPA) and alveolar haemorrhage.

HRCT: Nodules ± cavitation, pulmonary haemorrhage, reticulonodular patterns, peripheral wedge like consolidation (all GPA), ground glass change, bronchial wall thickening (EGPA) and alveolar haemorrhage.

Routine blood tests: Anaemia, ↑EΦ (EGPA), renal failure, ↑ESR.

Serum ANCA: See Box and Table 2.12.

Table 2.12 Types of pulmonary vasculitis

	Clinical features	Pulmonary involvement	ANCA & autoantibodies
Small vessel			
Microscopic Polyangiitis (MPA)	Most commonly *renal* (e.g. haematuria, proteinuria)	Frequently (≈ 50% of cases) → haemoptysis, haemorrhage, pleurisy or asthma	p-ANCA (c-ANCA often ↑)
Granulomatosis with Polyangiitis (GPA; Wegener's)	*ENT* disease (e.g. epistaxis, septum perforation, congestion, sinusitis, otitis, saddle nose). *Renal* (e.g. haematuria, proteinuria, red cell casts, renal failure). ↑T°, Wt loss, rash, joint pain, conjunctivitis, scleritis, proptosis, mononeuritis multiplex	Frequently (≈ 90% of cases) → flitting cavitating nodules, consolidation, haemoptysis, haemorrhage, pleurisy	c-ANCA (> 75%): levels correlate with disease severity/activity (may have role in monitoring). p-ANCA (10%): ANCA can be negative (often if disease confined to lung)
Eosinophilic Granulomatosis with Polyangiitis (EGPA; Churg–Strauss)	Typically asthma + blood eosinophilia (> 10% also ↑ in tissues) + features of systemic vasculitis: mononeuritis multiplex, sinus disease, cardiac (e.g. myositis), GI disturbance, ↑T°, Wt loss, rash, joint pain. See Box for differential diagnosis	Frequently → late-onset asthma (poorly controlled), flitting peripheral infiltrates, consolidation	p-ANCA (70%)

(Continued)

Table 2.12 Types of pulmonary vasculitis *(Continued)*

	Clinical features	Pulmonary involvement	ANCA & autoantibodies
Goodpasture's Disease	Renal (glomerulonephritis)	Frequently (≈ 90% of cases) → haemoptysis (smokers highest risk), patchy airspace shadows	Anti-glomerular basement membrane (GBM) p-ANCA (15%)
Medium vessel			
Polyarteritis Nodosa (PAN)	Similar to MPA. May overlap with GPA or EGPA	Rarely	ANCA Negative
Large vessel			
Giant cell arteritis	Headache, scalp tenderness, jaw pain, amaurosis fugax	Rarely (≈ 10%) → mild e.g. cough	ANCA Negative
Takayasu's arteritis	Young women (often Asian), affects aorta	Frequently (but often silent). Can cause mild PHT.	ANCA Negative

Anti-GBM (Goodpasture's): Anti-basement membrane IgG autoAbs targeting collagen in alveoli and glomeruli.
Urine dipstick and MC&S: Proteinuria, haematuria and granular/red cell casts.
Lung function: Obstructive (e.g. EGPA) or restrictive (e.g. Goodpasture's) $\pm$ ↑KCO (alveolar haemorrhage).
Sinus imaging (plain XR $\pm$ CT): Bony destruction (usually GPA).
Bronchoscopy: Signs of inflammation (inc URT) and haemorrhage. BAL → ↑NΦ or ↑EΦ (EGPA).
Biopsy (of affected site, e.g. nasal, renal, lung, skin): Histological confirmation often required for definitive diagnosis. **NB:** disease may be patchy (transbronchial biopsy usually not diagnostic).
Angiography: For Takayasu's arteritis.

2.13.2 Differential diagnosis for eosinophilic granulomatosis with polyangiitis

The following can also cause CXR infiltrates $\pm$ blood eosinophilia:

 Asthma with ABPA
 Acute or Chronic eosinophilic pneumonia: Unknown aetiology (sputum/BAL ↑ EΦ; blood EΦ may be normal)
 Hypereosinophilic syndrome: Unknown aetiology (↑↑EΦ > 1.5×10^9/L)
 Löffler's syndrome (simple pulmonary eosinophilia): Parasitic infection (*Ascaris lumbricoides*, *Strongyloides* or hookworm)
 Tropical pulmonary eosinophilia: Hypersensitivity to larvae of filarial worms
 Drug-induced pulmonary eosinophilia: E.g. inhaled cocaine, methotrexate, NSAIDs, penicillin (for extensive list consult: http://www.pneumotox.com)

MANAGEMENT OF SMALL VESSEL VASCULITIDES

Also see page 182 for details of immunosuppressant agents.
ALWAYS initiate osteoporosis and PCP prophylaxis where
appropriate! The following is a guide only (use local protocols
where available).

GPA (Wegener's)/MPA: Involve renal team early. **Suggested
Rx regimen:** (1) *Induce remission* (3–6 months Rx) with
prednisolone po (1 mg/kg/day; tapering dose as patient improves)
+ cyclophosphamide po (2 mg/kg/day) or iv (pulsed 3–4
wkly; 15 mg/kg). (2) *Maintain remission* (long-term Rx) with
prednisolone (usually ≤ 10 mg po) + azathioprine (usually 2 mg/kg/
day; can reduce after 1 yr) *or* methotrexate (azathioprine preferred;
usually methotrexate where ↓TPMT or SE). Rx is for several years
– monitor clinical state and ANCA. (3) *Relapse* on Rx (≈ 50%
patients) requires either ↑prednisolone dose (non-severe) or a repeat
induction of remission if severe (discussed earlier). (4) Options
for **severe or life-threatening disease** (e.g. rapidly progressive
RF or pulmonary haemorrhage) include: plasma exchange,
pulsed iv methylprednisolone (500 mg–1 g/day for 3 days) + iv
cyclophosphamide (discussed earlier) and dialysis. (5) **Refractory
disease** requires specialist input and consideration of infliximab,
rituximab, alemtuzumab and IV immunoglobulin.

Goodpasture's: Involve renal team early. **Suggested Rx
regimen:** (1) *Plasma exchange* (plasmapheresis) to remove anti-
GBM autoAbs and ↑ response to immunosuppression (usually
2–3 wks; until clinical improvement/undetectable anti-GBM).
(2) *Immunosuppressants* (as discussed earlier). May also require
dialysis ± renal transplantation (only if low anti-GBM). Once
controlled, recurrence is unusual and responds to Rx.

EGPA (Churg–Strauss) – Suggested Rx regimen: (1) *Induce
remission*–use prednisolone po alone (1 mg/kg) for *isolated
non-severe lung disease*. Use 3 days pulsed methylprednisolone iv
(discussed earlier) initially followed by prednisolone po +
cyclophosphamide (discussed earlier) for *severe cases or alveolar
haemorrhage*; (2) *maintain remission* with prednisolone po + one
other immunosuppressant (usually azathioprine). Isolated lung

disease has a good prognosis. Anti-interleukin-5 monoclonal antibodies (e.g. Reslizumab [CINQAERO]) are used in some centres.

SARCOIDOSIS

Multi-system disease characterised by *non-caseating granulomata*. Most commonly involves lungs ± associated lymph nodes (Box 2.14.1). But other organs can be affected (discussed hereunder). Unknown aetiology; likely abnormal immunological response to environmental triggers ± genetic susceptibility → CD4+ T-cell Th1-biased response. Incidence ≈ 10/100,000; commoner in black Africans or West Indians (↑ aggressive/worse prognosis) and Irish. Usually presents between ages 20 and 40. Many patients (> 50%) will spontaneously remit, but some develop chronic and progressive sarcoid.

2.14.1 Bilateral hilar lymphadenopathy (BHL)

Classical feature: Can be asymptomatic or cause cough ± chest pain. May be associated with systemic Sxs, e.g. malaise, fever or arthralgia. CT and lymph node biopsy/aspiration (EBUS or mediastinoscopy) may be required to exclude other possible causes, e.g. TB, lymphoma, lung cancer, fungal infection (coccidioidomycosis/histoplasmosis), mycoplasma, inorganic dusts (berylliosis/silicosis) and hypersensitivity pneumonitis.

PULMONARY SARCOIDOSIS

Most common manifestation (> 90%). Asymptomatic in ≈ 1/3rd, spontaneous remission in ≈ 2/3rd and < 1/3rd will have chronic disease. Consider as two distinct processes: (1) Löfgren's syndrome: acute and self-limiting (usually < 2 yrs) with fever, BHL, EN and arthralgia. (2) Infiltrative lung disease: more insidious, often persistent and progressive fibrosis (but may be asymptomatic or remit; "burnt out"). Pulmonary sarcoid can be staged according to CXR (*Scadding classification*): **Stage 0:** Normal, **Stage I:** hilar lymphadenopathy only (usually bilateral and symmetrical), **Stage II:** hilar lymphadenopathy + parenchymal infiltration, **Stage III:** parenchymal infiltration, **Stage IV:** fibrosis.

Investigations

Diagnosis based on characteristic clinical findings, HRCT ± histology (non-caseating granulomata) from any affected organ (**NB:** extra-thoracic may be easier to access). **Important:** ensure TB and lymphoma excluded! Some important investigations include:

FBC: Lymphopenia (↑Lɸ migration to lungs). ↓Hb, ↓Nɸ and ↓Plt less common.

U&E: ↑if renal involvement (discussed hereunder).

Calcium: Often ↑with active disease.

Serum ACE: Commonly raised (**NB:** suppressed by steroids). Useful marker of disease (↓with resolution). *Remember:* may still be normal with active disease and is not specific (e.g. ↑in TB).

Lung function: Can be normal, restrictive if lung fibrosis (+ ↓TLCO) or less commonly obstructive (e.g. airway involvement). Useful for monitoring disease progression/response to Rx.

CXR: See Scadding classification discussed earlier.

HRCT: Vast range of changes including: hilar and mediastinal lymphadenopathy, nodules, micronodules (may mimic miliary), larger opacities and fibrosis ± honeycombing (usually upper lobes with hyperinflation of lower lobes and raised hila).

Bronchoscopy: Only required if diagnostic doubt. Sampling can be via bronchoalveolar lavage (lymphocytosis) or bronchial biopsy (usually only if a visibly abnormal mucosa). Transbronchial biopsy is usually performed in conjunction with lymph node aspiration, often by endobronchial ultrasound (EBUS); dual sampling offers highest diagnostic yield! **NB:** there are several other causes of non-caseating granulomata (less common): atypical tuberculosis, berylliosis, carcinomatosis, drug reaction, eosinophilic granuloma, foreign body reaction, granulomatous arteritis, hypogammaglobulinaemia, fungal infection, biliary cirrhosis, cat scratch, leprosy, NTM infection, lymphoma, hypersensitivity pneumonitis, Q fever, syphilis, dialysis, GPA, histiocytosis-X, yaw and zirconium exposure.

Mediastinoscopy: Performed if diagnostic uncertainty or non-diagnostic bronchoscopy. Surgical biopsy (usually by video-assisted thoracoscopic surgery [VATS]) is rarely needed.

Mantoux/Heaf test: Rarely performed. Typically grade 0 in sarcoid (cutaneous anergy to tuberculin).

Management

Most patients with pulmonary sarcoid do NOT need Rx: especially asymptomatic or stable stage I, II or III disease. It can be difficult however to decide if disease is stable: use combination of Sx, radiology, lung function, serum ACE or Ca^{2+}. **Important:** look for presence of extra-thoracic disease (can determine if Rx is required; discussed hereunder Box 2.14.2).

2.14.2 Indications to start treatment for sarcoidosis

1 Progressive disease
2 Specific extra-thoracic involvement: cardiac, neurological, ocular (sight-threatening), splenic, hepatic or renal
3 ↑Ca^{2+}
4 Lupus pernio

Oral corticosteroids: Mainstay of Rx; usually prednisolone po. Start 0.5 mg/kg/day (max 40 mg) for 4 wks, then ↓ to maintenance dose (i.e. lowest dose that controls Sx and prevents progression; usually ≈ 5–10 mg). Identifying the optimum maintenance dose is tricky: wean slowly and re-assess. Maintenance Rx is usually required for prolonged period ≈ 1–2 yrs. Rarely required for longer; use 2.5–5 mg and consider steroid-sparing agents (discussed hereunder). Relapses may occur when weaning or stopping. Remember: bisphosphonate and PPI!

Inh corticosteroids: Limited efficacy and never in isolation. May be helpful for endobronchial sarcoid or cough.

IV methylprednisolone: Reserved for life-/organ-threatening disease.

Other immunosuppressants: Rarely required. Reserved for disease refractory to steroids, intolerable steroid SEs or steroid-sparing if prolonged Rx. 1st line is a 6–12 month-trial of methotrexate (10–15 mg po. Azathioprine 100–150 mg od po and hydroxychloroquine 200 mg od/bd po (esp if skin or $\uparrow$Ca^{2+}) are also occasionally used. Specialist centres occasionally use leflunomide, ciclosporin, thalidomide or TNF-α inhibitors.

Transplantation: Rare indication. Consider for end-stage lung fibrosis and rapidly progressive sarcoid.

EXTRATHORACIC SARCOIDOSIS

May have systemic non-specific Sxs e.g. $\uparrow$T$^{\circ}$, sweats, loss of appetite, Wt loss, fatigue and malaise. Specific features include:

$\uparrow$Ca^{2+}: Conversion of vit D3 $\to$ active 1,25 dihydroxycholecalciferol. May cause Sxs and renal damage. Advise limited dietary intake, hydration and avoiding sun exposure.

Cardiac: Most often conduction defects from myocardial granulomata (inc sudden death). Less commonly cardiac failure, valve disease, pericarditis and aneurysm. **NB:** perform regular screening ECGs in sarcoid. Biopsy may be required. Always Rx with po prednisolone. Consider arrhythmic drugs, PPM/ICD or transplantation.

Renal: Granulomata in the interstitium, nephrocalcinosis and nephrolithiasis. Always Rx with steroids and hydroxychloroquine for $\uparrow$Ca^{2+}.

Neural: Any part of PNS or CNS. May be non-specific or features of hypothalamic disease (e.g. DI). $\uparrow$ACE and $\uparrow$Lϕ in CSF. May require biopsy. Often resistant to steroids; consult specialist regarding alternative immunosuppressants (discussed earlier).

Skin: Erythema nodosum, lupus pernio, maculopapular rash, nodules, plaques and alopecia.

Eyes: Uveitis, episcleritis, scleritis, glaucoma, conjunctivitis and retinal involvement ($\downarrow$acuity/blindness). Can trial local steroids. But start parental Rx (discussed earlier) if sight at risk!

Musculoskeletal: Arthralgia, arthritis, proximal myopathy and bone cysts.
Hepatic: Usually asymptomatic. Rarely fibrosis and cirrhosis.
Splenomegaly: Can be massive and painful.
ENT: Granulomata of nasal/sinus cavities, larynx, parotid and salivary glands.
Rare: Testicular, ovarian or breast granulomata.

TUBERCULOSIS

MYCOBACTERIUM TUBERCULOSIS (MTB)

Infection results from inhalation of airborne droplets containing MTB. Can be 1° (Sx after initial inhalation), latent (LTB; inactive; no Sx) or 'post-1°' (reactivation of latent MTB). Host immunity plays an important role in MTB containment and reactivation. Most cases present with pulmonary MTB (inc pleural effusion, abscess, hilar lymphadenopathy and disseminated miliary MTB). Extrapulmonary cases account for ≈ 20%: CNS (inc meningitis), pericardial, spinal and renal.

Always have a low suspicion – MTB is "the great imitator"!

Diagnosis confirmed by identifying MTB within respiratory (e.g. sputum or BAL) or non-respiratory samples. Patients can be **smear positive** (Acid-fast bacilli [AFB] after ZN stain are seen on smear; most infectious!) or **culture positive** (AFB not seen on smear, but MTB subsequently grown on culture). **NB:** conventional culture can take 6 wks (MTB divides slowly). A diagnosis can also be made from classical caseating granulomas on **biopsy** (e.g. LN from EBUS or mediastinoscopy). **Nucleic acid amplification techniques** (confirm MTB serotype and drug susceptibility; e.g. Xpert® MTB/RIF) and **adenosine deaminase testing** are increasingly available. **Tuberculin skin tests** (**TST**; Mantoux) and Interferon-γ Release Assays (**IGRAs**; T-SPOT® or QuantiFERON®) are important in the diagnosis of LTB but cannot differentiate active MTB (see LTB; as discussed).

2.15.1 *Important points regarding treatment*

Always:

1 Involve respiratory team and specialist nurse (ensure contactable key worker)
2 Manage as OP wherever possible
3 Isolate suspected cases in negative pressure side-room (pulmonary TB)
4 Send samples for AFB/MC&S prior to Rx
5 Start Rx before results of culture and sensitivities BUT ONLY if MTB highly suspected
6 Notify all confirmed cases (even after death)
7 Check and document baseline LFTs/U&Es and visual acuity
8 Rx with combination of drugs (*always* > 1), over a long term and monitor for signs of poor compliance: MTB can naturally become resistant
9 Consider Directly Observed Therapy (DOT), if poor compliance or MDR-TB
10 Consider potential for drug interactions (esp HAART)
   — Standard Rx for MTB is 6 months: 2 months with 4 drugs and 4 months with 2 drugs
   — Rx for CNS involvements is 12 months
   — Doses are weight dependent and may require adjustment during Rx (discussed hereunder)
   — Nutritional supplementation should be considered
   — Corticosteroids are occasionally useful for pleural effusions, pericardial and CNS disease

Treatment (Box 2.15.1)

First line: THINK 'RIPE' **R**ifampicin, **I**soniazid, **P**yrazinamide and **E**thambutol. Patients at ↑ risk of drug-related neuropathy → pyridoxine 10 mg od po. Rx comes as individual or combination tablets (better compliance); Rifinah 150/100 (rifampicin 150 mg + isoniazid 100 mg), Rifinah 300/150 (rifampicin 300 mg + isoniazid 150 mg) or Rifater (rifampicin 120 mg + isoniazid 50 mg + pyrazinamide 300 mg) or Voractiv (ethambutol 275 mg, isoniazid 75 mg, pyrazinamide 400 mg, rifampicin 150 mg.

Initial 2 months: 'RIPE' (i.e. all four drugs). **Subsequent 4 months (or longer if infection CNS): 'RI'** (i.e. rifampicin + isoniazid). **Pregnancy:** the standard regimen is NOT teratogenic and can be used. Long-term follow-up is not required for compliant patients who improved on Rx. If a clinical response is not satisfactory, re-check sputum cultures prior to discontinuing Rx. Relapse is uncommon and usually from the same fully sensitive organism (use the same regimen). **DOT:** patients who cannot reliably comply with the above regimen should be considered for supervised drug administration (Directly Observed Therapy; **DOT**). Use 'RIPE' but 3 times/wk for first 2 months, followed by 'RI' 3 times/wk for a further 4 months Table 2.13.

Drug-resistant MTB

MTB resistant to 1 first-line anti-MTB agent. Unusual in the UK (but ↑ prevalence) and more common among non-Caucasians and HIV. Always involve senior specialist with MTB experience. In general, Rx must inc ≥ two drugs to which MTB is sensitive (Table 2.14).

MULTIDRUG-RESISTANT TUBERCULOSIS (MDR-TB)

MTB resistant to ≥ 2 first-line agents (usually isoniazid + rifampicin). Successful Rx outcomes are reported as ≈ 50% worldwide. MDR-TB that is also resistant to fluoroquinolones and ≥ 1 of the second-line anti-MTB injectable drugs (kanamycin, capreomycin or amikacin) is termed extensively drug-resistant TB (XDR-TB). XDR-TB has a mortality approaching 100%.

Treatment

Always seek expert advice from specialists experienced in managing resistant cases. There is a panel of experts based in Liverpool who can provide advice by email: MDRTBservice@ lhch.nhs.uk. Rx is complex and second-line agents toxic and often ineffective. Generally, start Rx with ≥ 5 drugs to which MDR-TB is sensitive. Continue all agents until sputum cultures are negative. A further 18–24 months is then required with ≥ 3 drugs to which MDR-TB is sensitive (Table 2.15).

Table 2.13 First-line anti-MTB treatment and doses

Drug	Weight	Dose	Notes
Separate preparations			
Rifampicin	<50 kg	450 mg od po	↑P450, ↓s fx OCP (other contraception needed), red discolouration urine & tears
	≥50 kg	600 mg od po	
	*600–900 mg po 3 times/wk		
Isoniazid	–	300 mg od po	↓P450, hepatitis & peripheral neuropathy (uncommon) → combine with 10 mg od po pyridoxine (diabetes, CKD, alcoholics, HIV)
		*15 mg/kg (max. 900 mg) po 3 times/wk	
Pyrazinamide	<50 kg	1.5 g od po	Hepatotoxic & GI upset
		*2 g po 3 times/wk	
	≥50 kg	2 g od po	
		*2.5 g po 3 times/wk	
Ethambutol	–	15 mg/kg od po	Neuritis: peripheral and optic (full eye examination prior to starting)
	–	*30 mg/kg po 3 times/wk	
Combination preparations			
RIFINAH	< 50 kg	3 tablets (150/100)	**Combine with pyrazinamide + ethambutol**
	≥ 50 kg	2 tablets (300/150)	
RIFATER	< 40 kg	3 tablets	**Combine with ethambutol**
	40–49 kg	4 tablets	
	50–64 kg	5 tablets	
	≥ 65 kg	6 tablets	
VORACTIV	< 40 kg	2 tablets	
	40–54 kg	3 tablets	
	55–70 kg	4 tablets	
	> 70 kg	5 tablets	

* Option for DOT.

Table 2.14 Examples of regimens for drug-resistant MTB

Resistance	Initial 2 months	Continuation phase
Isoniazid	Rifampicin + pyrazinamide + ethambutol	**7 months:** Rifampicin + pyrazinamide (10 months if extensive disease)
Pyrazinamide	Rifampicin + isoniazid + ethambutol	**7 months:** Rifampicin + isoniazid
Ethambutol	Rifampicin + isoniazid + pyrazinamide	**4 months:** Rifampicin + isoniazid
Rifampicin*	Isoniazid + pyrazinamide + ethambutol	**16 months:** Isoniazid + ethambutol

* Rifampicin mono-resistance is rare and usually indicates MDR-TB (Rx as MDR-TB until full sensitivities available).

Table 2.15 Examples of second-line anti-tuberculous drugs

Drug	Dose
Amikacin	15 mg/kg iv
Azithromycin	500 mg od po
Bedaquiline	400 mg od po for 2 wks; then 200 mg po 3 times/wk
Capreomycin	1g im od (max. 20 mg/kg)
Ciprofloxacin	750 mg bd po
Clarithromycin	500 mg od po
Clofazimine	100 mg od po
Cycloserine	250 mg bd po
Delamanid	100 mg bd po
Kanamycin	15 mg/kg iv
Levofloxacin	500 mg bd po
Linezolid	600 mg od po
Moxifloxacin	400 mg od po
Ofloxacin	400 mg bd po
Para-aminosalicylic acid (PAS)	4 g tds daily
Rifabutin	300–450 mg od po
Streptomycin	15 mg/kg iv
Thiacetazone	150 mg od po

MTB & HIV infection

Risk of developing MTB infection $\approx$ 30 times $\uparrow$ with HIV/AIDS. Four important to test all MTB patients for HIV. Involve HIV specialists early! Atypical presentations common if CD4 count < 200 $\times 10^6$/L, inc disseminated MTB with multi-organ involvement (inc bacteraemia) or asymptomatic disease. Generally start anti-MTB Rx before HIV Rx. HAART usually started < 8 wks of Rx $\rightarrow$ expect paradoxical worsening of Sx (immune reconstitution inflammatory syndrome). Anti-MTB regimens are the same, but avoid possible drug interactions (e.g. protease inhibitor with rifampicin)!

Latent TB infection

Defined as a persistent immune response to MTB (i.e. positive TST or IGRA) in the presence of a normal CXR and no Sxs of active MTB (Box 2.15.2). Represents a $\downarrow$number of organisms that are contained by host immunity. Latent MTB is *not* infectious. Lifetime risk of developing active MTB $\approx$ 5–10%. But $\uparrow$risk with immunosuppression, e.g. HIV, ESRF on HD, organ transplant, malignancy, anti-TNF-α therapy. Chemoprophylaxis significantly $\downarrow$s risk of subsequent active MTB development (below).

2.15.2 Tuberculin skin testing & interferon-γ release assays

No role in the diagnosis of active MTB (this requires AFB smear and culture)!

TST (Mantoux): Examines cell-mediated immunity to MTB. Intradermal injection of standard dose of tuberculin units $\rightarrow$ read reaction after 48–72 hours. Graded as: *negative* (< 5 mm), *positive* (5–14 mm) or **strongly positive** (> 14 mm). Interpretation depends on patient risk factors, e.g. significance when > 5 mm if HIV or > 14 mm if no MTB risk factors.

Interpret with caution: cross-reactivity with BCG, false negatives in immunocompromised (e.g. HIV, steroid use) and false positives with touching/scratching, allergy/hypersensitivity or NTM infection (see below).

IGRA (QuantiFERON-TB Gold or T-SPOT.TB): Detection of IFN-γ release from T-lymphocytes in response to MTB-specific antigens. More sensitive than TST for latent MTB (i.e. negative or↓ result rules out latent MTB). It can also distinguish between latent MTB and previous BCG/most NTM. However, it cannot differentiate between active and latent MTB.

Contact tracing

Undertaken for all active pulmonary and laryngeal MTB cases, even smear negative. NOT required for extra-pulmonary/laryngeal MTB. Close household contacts are traced for the period the index case was infectious *or* for 3 months prior to the first positive culture (if infectious period unknown). **Involves:** history, examination, CXR, TST ± IGRA and advice to report any Sx. Tracing will identify any transmitted cases of active infection (use standard Rx; discussed earlier), infection without evidence of active disease (consider chemoprophylaxis; discussed hereunder) and those suitable for BCG vaccination (discussed hereunder).

Immigrant screening

Immigrants account for > 70% of MTB cases in the UK. New entrants are four screened at port of arrival. Applications for all the UK visas (> 6 months) from residents of countries where MTB is common (> 40/100,000) will require screening at an approved centre. Screening can detect active MTB (standard Rx; discussed earlier), latent MTB (consider chemoprophylaxis; discussed hereunder) or those suitable for BCG vaccination (discussed hereunder).

Chemoprophylaxis

Given to MTB contacts or screened immigrants with latent MTB who display a positive IGRA or TST (strongly positive if prior BCG), but no clinical or radiological evidence of active MTB infection. There is always a risk of adverse effects from MTB drugs and a proportion of latent MTB might not develop into active MTB. *Chemoprophylaxis recommended for:* (1) < 35 yrs (↑risk of drug hepatotoxicity if older); (2) healthcare workers of any age; (3) any age of HIV patient (exclude active MTB first, esp if exposure to smear positive respiratory disease); (4) recent TST conversion (i.e. positive TST after a previously negative test); (5) evidence of previous MTB infection (e.g. CXR scar) without a history of adequate Rx; (6) with immunosuppression e.g. anti-TNF-α Rx.

Drug regimen

For patients without HIV: start either isoniazid for 6 months (↓risk of toxicity), rifampicin + isoniazid for 3 months *or* 6 months of rifampicin (if a contact of isoniazid-resistant disease). With HIV: use 6 months of isoniazid. Those who decline chemoprophylaxis should receive 'inform and advise' information regarding risks and Sx and be followed up at 3 and 12 months with a CXR.

BCG VACCINATION

Live attenuated vaccine. UK schools' vaccination programme has now ceased. Vaccination only offered to 'at risk' groups, e.g.:

- Infants with parents/grandparents originating from an area of ↑MTB incidence (> 40/100,000).
- Previously unvaccinated healthcare workers who are TST negative (other ↑ risk occupations can also be considered, e.g. care home worker, prison staff).
- Previously unvaccinated contacts of respiratory MTB patients who are TST negative (if aged < 35 yrs).
- Previously unvaccinated immigrants (aged < 16 yrs) from ↑ incidence areas (> 40/100,000). Those from sub-Saharan Africa or a country of very ↑ incidence (> 500/100,000) are vaccinated if < 35 yrs.

NB: adverse effects of vaccination include pain, suppuration at the injections site and localised lymphadenitis (3–6 month course of rifampicin ± isoniazid may be needed). ☠ Contraindicated if HIV positive (screen first if HIV suspected or patient is ↑risk) ☠.

NON-TUBERCULOUS MYCOBACTERIA (NTM)

Also known as atypical mycobacteria. Many different species but *Mycobacterium avium* complex (MAC), *M. kansasii*, *M. malmoense*, *M. abscessus* and *M. xenopi* are most important. They are environmental and low-grade pathogens causing pulmonary infection in susceptible individuals (e.g. immunocompromised, pre-existing lung disease or long-term macrolide use). Sx often non-specific (e.g. deteriorating respiratory state). Diagnosis made from AFB stain and subsequent NTM culture in respiratory samples ± suggestive clinical features (e.g. upper lobe cavitation, cylindrical bronchiectasis, tree-in-bud pattern or granulomatous histology). Often challenging to differentiate contamination and active infection. Good practice to send > 1 sample if NTM suspected/cultured and ONLY start Rx if consistently cultured.

Treatment

Rx is long term (usually 12–24 months) and carries ↑ risk of side effects. Only commence Rx when active infection is clinically suspected and ≥ 2 positive NTM cultures. Laboratory resistance does not always correlate with clinical response. **ALWAYS** involve microbiology, respiratory team and consult BTS guidance (https://www.brit-thoracic.org.uk/guidelines-and-quality-standards/non-tuberculous-mycobacteria/). Rx involves multiple drugs inc rifampicin 450 mg (< 50 kg) or 600 mg (≥ 50 kg) od po, ethambutol 15 mg/kg od po, isoniazid 300 mg od po and macrolides (clarithromycin or azithromycin). Always beware drug interactions (esp HAART Rx)! *M. abscessus* is a major pathogen in CF and is resistant to anti-MTB medication. It requires IV Rx (4 wks) with amikacin + imipenem + tigecycline (+ po clarithromycin/azithromycin) before long-term amikacin nebs, azithromycin po + 1–3 of clofazimine, linezolid, minocycline/doxycycline, quinolone (e.g. ciprofloxacin) and co-trimoxazole depending on S and tolerances.

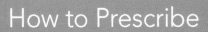

How to Prescribe

DOI: 10.1201/9781315151816-3

ANTICOAGULANTS

WARFARIN

Consult your local anticoagulant service if unsure about indications, doses or interactions. Refer as early before discharge as practicable so outpatient monitoring is arranged in time.

Basics

Oral anticoagulant for long-term Rx/Px of TE: loading (discussed hereunder) usually takes several days and is initially prothrombotic, so heparin or an LMWH, which is effective immediately, is used as short-term cover until therapeutic levels are achieved.

Monitoring & length of treatment

Via INR = ratio of patient's PT (prothrombin time) to a control raised to the power of a variable dependent on exact reagents used in each lab. A target INR is set at the start of Rx, according to indication (discussed hereunder); variations of $\pm$ 0.5 are acceptable. **NB:** for PE $\rightarrow$ target INR = 2.5; Rx is for 3 months (provoked) or 6 months/lifelong (unprovoked or if permanent risk factors). However, remember not ALL PE resolve within 6 months; therefore, if clot is large or patient remains symptomatic $\rightarrow$ reassess for residual PE (e.g. CTPA) and consider continuing warfarin.

Starting RX (for acute thrombosis)

Check INR before 1st dose and every day for 4 days, then assess stability of INR and adjust accordingly. If on LMWH, do not stop until 2 days after therapeutic INR achieved. For loading regimens, where possible use your hospital's own guidelines, since these often vary. Otherwise, it is sensible to use the BCSH guidelines (Table 3.1).

Table 3.1 BCSH guidelines for target INRs

Indication	Target INR ($\pm$ 0.5)
DVT/PE [1]	2.5
Thrombophilia (if symptomatic)[2]	2.5
Paroxysmal nocturnal haemoglobinuria (PNH)[3]	2.5
AF[4] (or other causes of cardiac emboli[5])	2.5
Bioprosthetic heart valves[6]	2.5
Mechanical heart valves[7]	3.5

Source: Adapted with permission from British Journal of Haematology 2011; 154(3): 311–24.

[1] Rx for = 6 wks if calf vein thrombosis; for = 3 months if provoked proximal (peroneal or above) DVT/PE; for = 6 months or lifelong if idiopathic venous TE or permanent risk factors. If recurrent DVT/PE whilst on therapeutic Rx, target INR = 3.5. Discuss all other than 1st presentation with anticoagulant service.

[2] Arterial thrombosis in antiphospholipid syndrome is exception with target INR 3.5.

[3] Paroxysmal nocturnal haemoglobinuria (PNH); only under guidance of consultant haematologist.

[4] Maintain INR > 2.0 for 3 wks before and 4 wks after elective DC cardioversion.

[5] Dilated cardiomyopathy, mural thrombus post-MI or rheumatic valve disease.

[6] Only for first 3–6 months post-valve insertion at discretion of each centre.

[7] For new generation aortic valves INR target 3.0.

Although not yet in the BCSH guidelines, a target INR of 2.5 is widely agreed for nephrotic syndrome (generally once albumin < 20 g/L).

NB: Slow loading with 3–5 mg for 5–7 days achieves therapeutic levels with less overshoot and may be preferable for outpatient initiation in atrial fibrillation (BCSH guidelines, 3rd edition, 2005 update: www.bcshguidelines.com).

If interrupting warfarin (e.g. before operation/procedure), assess thrombotic risk and use bridging anticoagulation with LMWH as necessary; do not reload postoperative as discussed earlier, but restart at usual dose +50% for 2 days, then return to usual dose *if no contraindications* (e.g. bleeding/taking **W+** drugs).

Warfarin and invasive procedures

Warfarin is often stopped 4–5 days ahead of surgery and other invasive procedures ($\pm$ heparin cover until day of procedure). Exact

Table 3.2 Warfarin loading regimen

Day 1		Day 2		Day 3		Day 4	
INR	Dose (mg)	INR	Dose (mg)	INR	Dose (mg)	INR	Dose¹ (mg)
< 1.4	10	< 1.8	10	< 2.0	10	< 1.4	> 8
		1.8	1	2.0–2.1	5	1.4	8
		> 1.8	0.5	2.2–2.3	4.5	1.5	7.5
				2.4–2.5	4	1.6–1.7	7
				2.6–2.7	3.5	1.8	6.5
				2.8–2.9	3	1.9	6
				3.0–3.1	2.5	2.0–2.1	5.5
				3.2–3.3	2	2.2–2.3	5
				3.4	1.5	2.4–2.6	4.5
				3.5	1	2.7–3.0	4
				3.6–4.0	0.5	3.1–3.5	3.5
				> 4.0	0	3.6–4.0	3
						4.1–4.5	Miss 1 day then 2 mg
						> 4.5	Miss 2 days then 1 mg

Source: Adapted with permission of BMJ group from Fennerty A, et al. BMJ 1984; 288: 1268–70.
¹ Predicted maintenance dose.

protocol depends on procedure involved and risks of bleeding versus thrombosis: get senior advice from team doing the procedure and haematologists if at all unsure.

For bronchoscopy: Warfarin is stopped 5 days before[BTS] and the INR checked (< 1.5 considered safe). It can be restarted at the usual dose on the evening of the bronchoscopy, provided significant bleeding is not anticipated. LMWH is used as 'cover' for high-risk patients (e.g. prosthetic metal MV, AF with MS or heart valve, < 3 months after VTE or thrombophilia); start 2 days after stopping warfarin, omit on day of bronchoscopy and continue until INR therapeutic.

3.1.1 Situations when doses (especially loading) may need review

↓**doses if:** Age > 80 yrs, LF, HF, postoperative, poor nutrition, ↑baseline INR or taking drugs that potentiate warfarin (check for **W+** symbols in this book) including almost all antibiotics.

↑**doses if:** Taking drugs that inhibit warfarin (check for **W−** symbols in this book).

Herbal remedies/non-prescription drugs: Can have significant interactions – always ask patients directly if taking any, as they may not realise the importance (e.g. glucosamine can ↑INR). Check each one with your hospital's drug information office for significance.

Alcohol and diet: Can affect dosing, especially if intake varies – the goalposts will move for an individual's therapeutic range. It is a common misconception that BMI influences response.

Make small infrequent dose changes unless INR dangerously high or low. 'Steering a supertanker' is a good analogy; there is often significant delay between dose changes and their fx.

Warfarin and pregnancy

Warfarin is contraindicated in early pregnancy (teratogenic during weeks 6–12). Women of childbearing age must be counselled by a specialist prior to planning pregnancy (inc informed to do pregnancy test whenever a period is > 2 days late) and any woman who is pregnant and on warfarin must be converted immediately to

---

3.1.2 Overtreatment/poisoning

Seek expert help from haematology on-call as xs vitamin K can make re-anticoagulation difficult, as fx can last for weeks; therefore, ⇒ ↑risk from condition that warfarin was started for.

Table 3.3 Recommendations for Mx of excess warfarin (BCSH guidelines)

INR	Action
3.0–6.0 if target 2.5 (4.0–6.0 if target 3.5)	↓dose or stop warfarin; restart when INR < 5.0
6.0–8.0 and no/minor bleeding	Stop warfarin; restart when INR < 5.0
> 8.0 and no/minor bleeding	Stop warfarin; restart when INR < 5.0
	If other bleeding risks (e.g. age > 70 yrs, Hx of bleeding complications *or* liver disease) give phytomenadione (vit K$_1$) 0.5 mg[1] iv or 5 mg po
Major bleeding, e.g. ↓ing Hb or cardiodynamic instability	Stop warfarin Phytomenadione (vit K$_1$) 5 or 10 mg iv, repeating 24 h later, if necessary Prothrombin complex concentrate 25–50 units/kg not exceeding 3000 units (if unavailable give FFP[2] 15 mL/kg)

Source: Adapted with permission from British Journal of Haematology 2011; 154(3): 311–24.

[1] Since the publication of the BCSH guidelines some clinicians advise larger doses of iv vit K, e.g. 2 mg.

[2] Although not stated in the BCSH guidelines, it should be noted that FFP is not fully effective at warfarin reversal.

LMWH under specialist guidance. Rx for PE in pregnant patients = LMWH until at least 6 wks after deliver.

DIRECT ORAL ANTICOAGULANTS (DOACs)

DOACs (Dabigatran, Rivaroxaban, Apixaban and Edoxaban) are now licensed for the Rx of DVT and PE[NICE]. The length of Rx is 3–6 months (see Warfarin discussed earlier). They are also given for extended thromboprophylaxis after elective total knee or hip replacement[NICE] and for prevention of stroke and other systemic embolism in non-valvular AF[NICE]. **NB**: DOACs that inhibit factor Xa contain X in the name (e.g. Rivaro**X**aban, Api**X**aban and Edo**X**aban).

- **Dabigatran etexilate** (Pradaxa): Direct thrombin inhibitor. Dose for Rx of DVT and PE = 150 mg bd following > 5 days parental anticoagulation; use 110 mg with older patients, concomitant verapamil, renal impairment or ↑risk of bleeding. The same dosing is used for the prophylaxis of recurrent DVT and PE. **NB:** avoid if LF (esp if prolonged PT) or GFR < 30 mL/min. **VITAL:** Idarucizumab (Praxbind) is a monoclonal antibody fragment that binds dabigatran (+ metabolites) and reverses its anticoagulant effects (single 5 g ivi followed by further dose if required).

- **Rivaroxaban** (Xarelto): Direct inhibitor of activated factor Xa. Dose for Rx of DVT and PE = 15 mg bd (initial 21 days) then switch to 20 mg od. The same dosing is used for the prophylaxis of recurrent DVT and PE. **NB:** avoid if LF (esp if prolonged PT) or GFR < 15 mL/min.

- **Apixaban** (Eliquis): Direct inhibitor of activated factor Xa. Dose for Rx of DVT and PE = 10 mg bd (initial 7 days) then switch to 5 mg bd. 2.5 mg bd is used for the prophylaxis of recurrent DVT and PE. **NB:** avoid if LF (esp if prolonged PT) or GFR < 15 mL/min.

- **Edoxaban** (Lixiana): Direct inhibitor of activated factor Xa. Dose for Rx of DVT and PE = 30 mg od (60 mg of for > 60 kg). The same dosing is used for the prophylaxis of recurrent DVT and PE. **NB:** avoid if severe LF or ESRF/dialysis.

DOACs are attractive agents for the Rx of VTE, esp as they do not require INR monitoring and have fewer drug/food interactions compared to warfarin. ☠ However, there are no reversal agents in the event of bleeding or overdose (exception of Idarucizumab; discussed earlier), and they should not be used as alternatives to UF heparin in PE with haemodynamic instability, or those who may receive thrombolysis or embolectomy. ☠ **VITAL:** in the event of significant bleeding while on a DOAC, always consult haematology for advice as clotting factor replacement can be required (e.g. prothrombin complex concentrates).

HEPARIN

For immediate and short-term Rx/Px of TE. Two major types: low-molecular-weight heparins (LMWHs) and unfractionated (UF) heparin.

LMWHs

Given sc. ↑convenience (↓monitoring, can give to outpatients). ↓incidence of HIT* and osteoporosis cf unfractionated heparin means now preferred for many indications (e.g. MI/ACS, DVT/ PE Rx and pre-cardioversion of AF). Also Rx of choice for PE in patients with cancer. Caution in renal impairment, if severe consider using UF heparin.

Dalteparin (FRAGMIN), enoxaparin (CLEXANE) and tinzaparin (INNOHEP) are the most commonly used; each hospital tends to use one in particular; ask nurses which one they stock or call pharmacy. Prophylaxis does not need monitoring but do not use for > 7–10 days if creatinine > 150.

Monitoring of treatment with LMWH: Via peak anti-Xa assay: usually necessary only if renal impairment (i.e. creatinine > 150), pregnancy or at extremes of Wt (i.e. < 45 kg or > 100 kg). Take sample 3–4 h post-dose.

3.1.3 *HIT = Heparin-induced thrombocytopenia

Much more common with UF heparin but can occur with all heparins. Watch for ↓ing platelet count. Get senior help if concerned. Discuss investigation and Mx with haematologist. If HIT confirmed, stop heparin immediately – danaparoid (ORGARAN) or lepirudin (REFLUDAN) may be substituted.

Unfractionated heparin

Given iv: quickly reversible (immediately if protamine given; see page 156), which makes it useful in settings where desired amount of anticoagulation may change rapidly, e.g. perioperatively, patient at ↑risk of bleeding, or if using extracorporeal circuits such as cardiopulmonary bypass and haemodialysis. Can also be used with recombinant fibrinolytics thrombolysis of PE (or AMI). Due to difficulty keeping in therapeutic range, LMWH increasingly preferred where possible – discuss with senior if contemplating use.

Can be given sc (only for Px), but now largely replaced by LMWH.

Monitoring: Via APTT ratio (= **A**ctivated **P**artial **T**hromboplastin **T**ime of patient plasma divided by that of control plasma). Results can (rarely) be given as patient's exact APTT: the normal range is 35–45 sec. You then need to calculate the ratio: take the middle of the normal range for your lab (e.g. 40 sec) for your calculations. *Target ratio is commonly 1.5–2.5,* but this can vary: check your hospital's protocol and aim for the middle of range. **NB:** there is no national (let alone international) consensus on methods of measuring APTT, so results are not yet standardised.

Starting iv treatment:

1. *Load with 5000** units as iv bolus*: prescribed on the 'once-only' section of the drug chart (give 10,000** units if large or life-threatening PE).
2. Set up ivi at 15–25 units/kg/h: usually = 1000–2000 units/h. A sensible starting rate is 1500 units/h, which can be achieved by adding 25,000 units of heparin to 48 mL of normal saline to make 50 mL of solution (500 units/mL), which runs at 3 mL/h via a syringe driver. This can be written up as shown in Figure 3.1.

Check APTT ratio after 6 h, then 6–10 h until stable, and then daily at a minimum, adjusting to the following regimen (based on APTT *ratio* therapeutic range of 1.5–2.5; **NB:** *don't take sample from drip arm* [unless from site distal to ivi]).

Date/ Time	Infusion Fluid	Vol- ume	Additives If Any Drug and Dose	Rate of Admin	Dura- tion	Dr's Signature	Time Star- ted	Time Compl- eted	Set Up By Sig- nature	Batch No.
08/01	Normal saline	50 ml	HEPARIN 25,000 units			TN				
	Run at 3 ml per hour as ivi									

Figure 3.1 Drug chart showing how to write up heparin.

Table 3.4 APPT ratio and heparin doses

APTT ratio	Action
< 1.2	Give 5000-unit bolus iv and ↑ivi by 200–250 units/h
1.2–1.4	Give 2500-unit bolus iv and ↑ivi by 100–150 units/h
1.5–2.5	No change
2.6–3.0	↓ivi by 100–150 units/h
> 3.0	Stop ivi for 1 h then restart ivi, ↓ing by 200–250 units/h

Adjustments are safest made by writing a fresh ivi prescription at a different strength, but the same effect can also be achieved by calculating the appropriate rate change to the original prescription.

Variable rate of ivi (for fixed prescription of 25,000 units heparin in 50 mL saline) (Table 3.5):

Table 3.5 Variable rate of iv heparin infusion

Desired heparin ivi rate (units/h)	Rate of ivi (mL/h)	Desired heparin ivi rate (units/h)	Rate of ivi (mL/h)
1000	2.0	1500	3.0
1050	2.1	1550	3.1
1100	2.2	1600	3.2
1150	2.3	1650	3.3
1200	2.4	1700	3.4
1250	2.5	1750	3.5
1300	2.6	1800	3.6
1350	2.7	1850	3.7
1400	2.8	1900	3.8
1450	2.9	1950	3.9

Overtreatment/poisoning (LMWH and UF heparin): If significant bleeding, stop heparin and observe: iv heparin has short $t_{1/2}$ (30 min–2 h), so fx wear off quickly. If bleeding continues or is life-threatening, consider iv protamine (1 mg per 80–100 units of heparin to be neutralised as ivi over 10 min. ↓doses if giving >15 min after heparin stopped). **NB:** protamine is less effective against LMWH, and repeat administration may be required. Seek expert help from haematology on-call, if in any doubt!

FONDAPARINUX (ARIXTRA)

Parenteral anticoagulant (synthetic pentasaccharide) most commonly used in the Rx of MI/ACS. Also licensed for use for Rx and Px of VTE; useful with history of HIT* or allergy to heparin. Dose = 5 mg sc od (weight < 50 kg), 7.5 mg sc od (weight 50–100 kg) or 10 mg (weight > 100 kg). ☠Caution if RF or LF ☠.

CONTROLLED DRUGS

These drugs are rarely if ever prescribed to take home from the ED, except for severe acute pain or palliative care. **NB:** chronic users of controlled drugs should *only* receive new supplies from authorised/licensed medical practitioners.

  Note: Special 'Prescription requirements' apply in the UK to 'schedule' 1, 2 or 3 drugs only, the most likely of which might be prescribed by a junior doctor are morphine, diamorphine, fentanyl, methadone, oxycodone (and less commonly buprenorphine or pethidine). The following must be written 'so as to be indelible, e.g. written by hand, typed or computer generated' (**NB:** *this is a recent change from previously having to be written by hand – only the signature now needs to be handwritten*):

- Date.
- The patient's full name and address and, where appropriate, age.
- Drug name plus its form* (and, where appropriate, strength).
- Dosing regimen (**NB:** the directions 'take one as directed' constitutes a dose but 'as directed' does not).
- Total amount of drug to be dispensed in words and figures (e.g. for morphine 5 mg qds for 1 wk (5 mg 34 times a day 37 days = 140) write: '140 milligrams = one hundred and forty milligrams').
- Prescriber's address must be specified (should already be on prescription form, e.g. hospital address).

*Omitting the form (e.g. tablet/liquid/patch) is a common reason for an invalid prescription. It is often assumed to be obvious from the prescription (e.g. fentanyl as a patch or **Oramorph** as a liquid), but it still has to be written even if only one form exists.

These requirements *do not* apply to temazepam (despite being schedule 3), schedule 4 drugs (e.g. benzodiazepines) and schedule 5 drugs (such as codeine, dihydrocodeine/**DF118** and tramadol). For full details on controlled drug guidance in the UK, see www.dh.gov.uk/controlleddrugs.

INHALERS AND NEBULISERS

INHALERS

Cornerstone of Rx for airways disease (asthma and COPD). Vary in both drug content (*e.g.* SABA, SAMA, LABA, LAMA, ICS or combinations) AND type of device (discussed hereunder). Some are licensed for asthma or COPD exclusively, and some for both. Many different devices available, but essentially two main types: **metered dose inhaler** (**MDI**; either pressurised, i.e. **pMDI** or **breath-actuated MDI**) and **dry powder inhaler** (**DPI**). See Table 3.6 for advantages/disadvantages. **Soft mist inhalers** (**SMI**; RESPIMAT) are also available. They are propellant-free and deliver a metered dosage via a fine mist.

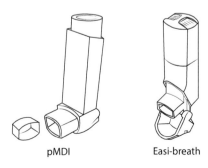

pMDI   Easi-breath

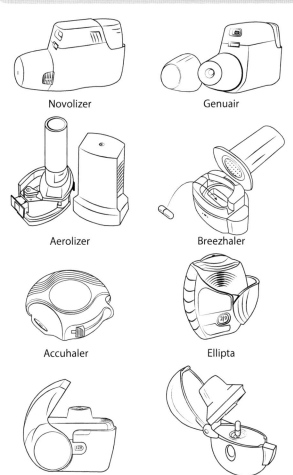

Novolizer

Genuair

Aerolizer

Breezhaler

Accuhaler

Ellipta

Nexthaler

Handihaler

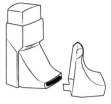

Clickhaler

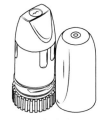

Turbohaler

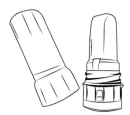

Twisthaler

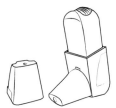

Easyhaler

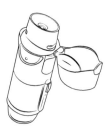

Respimat

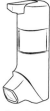

Autohaler

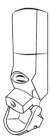

Spiromax

Table 3.6 Advantages and disadvantages of MDI and DPI inhalers

	Advantages	Disadvantages
MDI	• Drug is aerosolised and metered (i.e. dose and particle size is independent of inhalation manoeuvre) • Gentle inspiratory manoeuvre required • Most suitable for acutely SOB patients	• Coordination of inhalation and actuation required (unless breath-actuated or with spacer) • ↑oropharyngeal deposition (↓with spacer) • Requires propellant • No control of remaining doses
DPI	• Less patient coordination is required (breath-actuated)	• Requires forceful inspiratory manoeuvre to generate particles • Not suitable for acutely SOB patients • Affected by humidity

3.3.1 Prescribing inhalers – Top Tips

1 Before prescribing, ideally demonstrate inhaler technique and try a range of devices.
2 Patient preference may ↑adherence and drug delivery (e.g. convenience or ease of use).
3 Check inhaler technique at every opportunity and especially before uptitrating Rx (**NB:** poor clinical response may be secondary to poor inhaler technique).
4 If patient cannot manage a particular device → switch to another.
5 Spacer devices for MDIs can ↑lung delivery, ↓oropharyngeal deposition and help coordinate administration (esp children and elderly).
6 Ensure patient knows how to recognise that their device is empty (shake or dose counter).
7 Ensure patient carries a spare device/capsules, in case it runs out.
8 When switching inhaled drug (e.g. uptitrating or stepping down Rx), try to keep to the same device.
9 Combination inhalers may improve compliance.

10 When prescribing: use brand name and the same type of
   device for all the drugs used by a patient.
11 Counsel patient to rinse mouth, gargle with water or brush
   teeth and spit out residue (for ICS-containing inhalers to
   prevent oral candidiasis).

Guide to using different inhaler devices

A. pMDI
Example: EVOHALER
Instructions for pMDI:

1. May need to prime inhaler (if used for first time or not used for
   a while, e.g. > 5 days)
2. Remove cap from mouthpiece
3. Shake inhaler
4. Hold inhaler upright with thumb on base and first finger on
   metal canister
5. Exhale as far as is comfortable
6. Seal lips around mouthpiece (do not bite)
7. Start to inhale *slowly* through the mouth
8. Immediately activate inhaler by pressing the top of the canister
   with inhalation
9. Breathe in slowly and deeply, over at least 5 sec and until full
   inspiration
10. Hold at full inspiration for as long as possible, then relax
11. Replace the cap
12. Regularly check the dose counter on the inhaler (if it has one)
    to ensure it does not run out and keep a spare inhaler in case
13. Wait ≈ 30 sec until repeating for second dose
14. Wash inhaler every 2–3 wks

NB: Important *NOT* to: breathe in too quickly, activate inhaler
before inspiration, stop inhaling after activation or when drug is
tasted/felt in mouth.

Top Tip: pMDI are best used in conjunction with a spacer device: NEBUHALER, NEBUCHAMBER, VOLUMATIC, AERO CHAMBER, ABLE SPACER, PARI VORTEX SPACER, POCKET CHAMBER, OPTICHAMBER, OPTIHALER.

Instructions for pMDI with spacer device:

1. Ensure spacer is compatible with inhaler
2. Remove cap from mouthpiece
3. Shake inhaler
4. Insert mouthpiece into end of spacer device
5. Breath out as far as is comfortable
6. Seal lips around mouthpiece of spacer
7. Activate inhaler by pressing the top of the canister
8. Take one slow, deep breath in and hold at full inspiration for as long as possible, then relax *or* alternatively take three steady deep breaths in and out
9. Disconnect the device from spacer
10. Replace the cap
11. Clean spacer once a month with mild detergent, rinse and allow to air dry (avoids static charge). Replace spacer every 6–12 months

B. Breath-actuated MDI

Examples: AUTOHALER, EASI-BREATHE
Instructions for breath-actuated pMDI:

1. May need to prime inhaler (if used for first time or not used for a while, e.g. > 5 days)
2. Shake inhaler
3. Prepare device:
   a. EASI-BREATHE: Load inhaler by opening hinged cap
   b. AUTOHALER: Remove cap from mouthpiece and load inhaler by lifting lever
4. Always hold device upright
5. Breath out as far as is comfortable
6. Seal lips around mouthpiece (do not bite)
7. Inhale slowly and deeply, over at least 5 sec and until full inspiration

8. The device will click during inspiration: continue inhaling (**NB:** if a click is not heard then the device has not been activated → start again)
9. Hold at full inspiration for as long as possible, then relax
10. Replace the cap
11. Always keep a spare inhaler
12. To take a second dose the device must be reloaded by either lowering and raising the lever (AUTOHALER) or closing and reopening the cap (EASI-BREATHE)
13. EASI-BREATHE can be used with a spacer device (as discussed earlier), but it will need to be removed in between doses to allow the device to be reloaded

NB: Important *not* to: breathe in too quickly, stop inspiration when the click is heard, hold the device horizontally during use, stop inhaling after activation or when drug is tasted/felt in mouth.

C. DPI
Examples: ACCUHALER, TURBOHALER, HANDIHALER, CLICKHALER, TWISTHALER, EASYHALER, AEROLIZER, NOVOLIZER, BREEZHALER, DISCHALER, GENUAIR, PULVINAL, CYCLOHALER, AEROCAPS, ELLIPTA, SPIROMAX
Instructions for DPI:

1. Prime device (different for each; some examples are given here):
   a. ACCUHALER: Open device cover and push lever across until it clicks (pierces blister)
   b. TURBOHALER: With device in the upright position, unscrew cap and turn base forwards and backwards
   c. HANDIHALER/BREEZHALER/AEROLIZER: Open device, place capsule into chamber, close and pierce capsule by firmly pressing side buttons (keep in upright position)
   d. TWISTHALER: Remove cap by twisting
   e. NOVOLILIZER: Remove cap, press button and release when you hear a click (coloured window should change from red to green)

f. EASYHALER: Remove cap off and load in the vertical position while holding upright
g. NEXTHALER: Open cap until it clicks
h. ELLIPTA: Slide cap down until it clicks
i. SPIROMAX: Open cap and listen for click

2. Hold all DPIs level after priming
3. Exhale fully
4. Place DPI mouthpiece into mouth
5. Inhale deeply and forcefully until full inspiration (much faster than with MDI)
6. Hold breath at full inspiration for as long as possible
7. Repeat priming before taking a second dose

NB: Important *not* to: breathe in too slowly, hold the DPI horizontally during use, shake, blow into the device, swallow any capsules, leave cap off in between use, store in damp conditions or get the device wet.

D. SMI

Examples: RESPIMAT for SPIRIVA (tiotropium) or SPIOLTO

Instructions for SMI:

1. Insert canister into the device
2. Hold upright and turn the base until it clicks (with the cap remaining closed)
3. Flip open cap
4. Exhale and insert the mouthpiece, sealing tightly with lips (SMI should be pointing horizontally towards back of throat)
5. Press the button while inhaling, using a deep and slow breath
6. Hold breath in full inspiration (ideally 10 sec) before exhaling
7. For a second dose start by re-priming the device

NEBULISERS

Nebulisers use compressed air, O_2 (care/avoid if COPD!) or ultrasonic power to break up drug solutions or suspensions into small aerosol droplets for inhalation (Table 3.7). They can be used

Table 3.7 Some important nebulised drugs and important notes

Drug	Important notes
ß2 agonists (e.g. salbutamol, terbutaline) **Antimuscarinics** (e.g. ipratropium bromide)	• Also available as combination (COMBIVENT; salbutamol + ipratropium bromide) • Deliver ipratropium via mouthpiece (*not* face mask) to avoid glaucoma (atropine-like effects on eye)
Corticosteroids (e.g. budesonide, fluticasone)	• Viscous liquid → requires certain nebulisers • Administer via mouthpiece (*not* face mask) to avoid contact with eyes • Not compatible with other drugs (do *not* mix) • Encourage mouth rinses after to avoid oral candida • Thoroughly clean all equipment and do *not* reuse any disposables
Antibiotics (e.g. tobramycin, colomycin, amphotericin, ribavirin, pentamidine)	• Always use filtered system • Requires more powerful pump and special neb set • Best used with mouthpiece (*not* face mask) • May induce bronchoconstriction (administer first dose in hospital under supervision, with pre- and post-spirometry)
Saline	• Available as normal saline and hypertonic saline (3%, 6% and 7%) • Hypertonic saline may induce bronchoconstriction (administer first dose in hospital with pre- and post-spirometry)
RhDNase (e.g. PULMOZYME)	• For CF patients • Do *not* use ultrasonic nebuliser
Mannitol (e.g. BRONCHITOL)	• For CF patients if no improvement with saline/ RhDNase
Adrenaline	• For haemoptysis or upper airway obstruction • Use 1 mL of 1:1000 mixed with 4 mL of normal saline

for bronchodilators, corticosteroids, antibiotics, saline and some
other drugs (e.g. RhDNase, adrenaline).

**Principle reasons for selecting a nebuliser over an
inhaler include:** Disease severity, inability to use inhalers
and acute respiratory illness (consider MDI + spacer; can be as
effective). They do not require coordination, are effective with
tidal breathing, can be supplemented with O_2 and several drugs
can be administered together. **Disadvantages:** not very portable,
require time to prepare, administer and clean, and are expensive.
Always consider pros/cons and discuss with patient before
prescribing. NB: start with 2–4 wks trial and assess response
before a regular prescription.

Instructions for nebuliser:

1. Check drug compatibility (only mix compatible drugs).
2. Open ampoule(s) containing drug solution(s) or suspension(s)
   (do *not* use ultrasonic nebulisers for suspensions).
3. Squirt drug into chamber and attach to the face mask or
   mouthpiece (use mouthpiece rather than face mask for
   ipratropium bromide, corticosteroids and antibiotics). Some
   drugs require dilution (e.g. with sodium chloride 0.9%).
4. Place face mask over mouth and nose or position mouthpiece
   between lips.
5. Turn on compressor.
6. Inspire and expire slowly.
7. Use until nebulised solution has run out.
8. Switch off compressor.
9. Rinse/wash nebuliser chamber with hot water ± dilute
   washing-up liquid.
10. Dispose of any tubing and mouthpiece.
11. O_2 can be used with nebuliser either by wearing nasal
    prongs *or* by directly driving nebuliser with O_2 (i.e. attached
    to chamber). NB: most home O_2 cylinders do not provide
    sufficient flow rates for driving nebulisers.

INTRAVENOUS FLUIDS

The same degree of care should be taken when 'prescribing' intravenous fluids in the emergency department (ED) on the fluid order form, as when writing up drugs on the medication chart.

See Table 3.8 for the composition of the iv fluids most commonly used in the ED.

CRYSTALLOIDS

Isotonic: Used for replacement and/or maintenance regimens:

- **Normal (0.9%) saline:** One litre contains 154 mmol Na^+. Use as replacement and maintenance fluid in all situations, unless local protocol dictates otherwise. Caution in $\neq Na^+$ and liver dysfunction.
- **Hartmann's solution:** Compound sodium lactate used instead of normal saline (note 1 litre contains 5 mmol K^+). Avoid if RF.
- **Glucose* saline:** One litre contains mixture of NaCl (30 mmol Na^+) and glucose (4% = 222 mmol). Although considered useful as contains correct proportions of constituents (excluding KCl, which can be added to each bag) for 'average' daily requirements (see below), it will soon lead to hyponatraemia longer term (days), and does not account for individual patient needs. Also used as ivi in insulin sliding scales (see p. 205).
- **5% glucose*:** One litre contains 278 mmol (= 50 g) glucose, which is rapidly taken up by cells and included only to make the fluid isotonic (calories are minimal, at 200 kcal). Used as method of giving pure H_2O and as ivi with insulin sliding scales (see p. 205).

NB: commonest cause of $\varnothing Na^+$ in hospital is overuse of glucose saline or 5% glucose as fluid replacement (often postoperative).

Non-isotonic: Only for specialist/emergency situations by those experienced in their use:

- **Hypertonic (5%) saline:** One litre contains 856 mmol Na^+; given for severe symptomatic hyponatraemia, i.e. with seizures.
  ☠ Seek specialist help first ☠.
- **Hypotonic (0.45%) saline:** For severe $\neq Na^+$ (e.g. HHS).

Table 3.8 Composition of commonly used fluids

Composition of commonly used intravenous fluids

	Na (mmol/L)	Cl (mmol/L)	K (mmol/L)	Ca (mmol/L)	Mg (mmol/L)	Other constituents (/L)	Osmolarity mOsm/L (osmolality mOsm/kg)	pH
CRYSTALLOIDS								
0.9% sodium chloride (*normal saline*)	154	154	–	–	–	–	308 (300)	4.0–7.0
0.45% sodium chloride (*half normal saline*)	77	77	–	–	–	–	154 (150)	4.0–7.0
Hartmann's solution (*compound sodium lactate*)	131	111	5	2	–	29 mmol lactate	280 (274)	5.0–7.0
Modified Hartmann's	131	135	29.5	2	–	29 mmol lactate	329 (324)	
Ringer's lactate	130	109	4	3	–	28 mmol lactate	272	
5% dextrose	–	–	–	–	–	50 g dextrose	278 (252)	3.5–6.5
10% dextrose	–	–	–	–	–	100 g dextrose	556 (505)	3.5–6.5
50% dextrose	–	–	–	–	–	500 g dextrose	2778 (2525)	3.5–6.5
3.3% dextrose, 0.3% sodium chloride (*3 and a 1/3*)	51	51	–	–	–	33 g dextrose	286 (284)	3.5–6.5

(Continued)

Table 3.8 Composition of commonly used fluids (*Continued*)

Composition of commonly used intravenous fluids

	Na (mmol/L)	Cl (mmol/L)	K (mmol/L)	Ca (mmol/L)	Mg (mmol/L)	Other constituents (/L)	Osmolarity mOsm/L (osmolality mOsm/kg)	pH
4% dextrose, 0.18% sodium chloride (4 and a 1/5)	30	30	–	–	–	40 g dextrose	284 (282)	3.5–6.5
8.4% sodium bicarbonate	1000	–	–	–	–	1000 mmol HCO_3^-	–	–
Plasma-Lyte	140	98	5	–	1.5	27 mmol acetate 23 mmol gluconate	294 (294)	4.0–6.5
Plasma-Lyte– Replacement and Glucose 5%	140	98	5	–	1.5	27 mmol acetate 23 mmol gluconate 50 g dextrose	547 (573)	4.0–6.0
Plasma-Lyte Maintenance and 5% Glucose	40	40	13	–	1.5	16 mmol acetate 50 g dextrose	363 (389)	

(*Continued*)

Table 3.8 Composition of commonly used fluids (Continued)

Composition of commonly used intravenous fluids

	Na (mmol/L)	Cl (mmol/L)	K (mmol/L)	Ca (mmol/L)	Mg (mmol/L)	Other constituents (/L)	Osmolarity mOsm/L (osmolality mOsm/kg)	pH
COLLOIDS								
Gelofusine	154	120	–	–	–	40 g suc-cinylated gelatin	274	7.4+/– 0.3
Albumin 4%	140	128	< 2	–	–	40 g albumin 6.4 mmol octanoate		
Haemaccel	145	145	5.1	6.25	–	35 g Polygeline	301 (293)	7.3+/– 0.3
Dextran 40 in 0.9% Saline	150	150	–	–	–	Dextran 40 g	(325)	6.0
Dextran 40 in 5% Dextrose	–	–	–	–	–	Dextran 40 g dextrose 50 g	(349)	5.0
Dextran 70 in 0.9% Saline	150	150	–	–	–	Dextran 70 g	(306)	6.0
Dextran 70 in 5% Dextrose	–	–	–	–	–	Dextran 70 g dextrose 50 g	(325)	4.5

- **10%** and **20% glucose***: For mild/moderate hypoglycaemia.
- **50% glucose***: For severe hypoglycaemia (see p. 251), or if insulin being used to lower K$^+$ (see p. 269).
- **Sodium bicarbonate (1.26% or move rarely 1.4%)**: Useful replacement for 0.9% saline if ØpH or ≠K$^+$ which often coexist. Not isotonic so caution re: salt load and accompanying fluid retention ☠. Seek specialist help from nephrologists/others accustomed to its use ☠.

*NB: Glucose = dextrose. Low-strength glucose solutions used to be called dextrose solutions; this is now being phased out.

COLLOIDS
Plasma expanders and substitutes helpful to ≠/maintain plasma oncotic pressure.

- **Gelofusine:** Succinylated gelatin used in resuscitation of shock (non-cardiogenic). NB: electrolyte content is often overlooked: One litre **Gelofusine** has 154 mmol Na$^+$.
- **Albumin:** Prepared from whole blood and containing soluble proteins and electrolytes, but no clotting factors etc. May be fluid of choice in sepsis.
- **Haemaccel:** Bovine-derived polygeline (derivative of gelatin), may cause anaphylaxis.

DAILY FLUID AND ELECTROLYTE REQUIREMENTS (STANDARD)
Standard daily fluid and electrolyte requirement: For a 70-kg adult male is approximately 30–40 mL/kg H$_2$O (3 L); 1.5–2.0 mmol/kg Na$^+$ (100–150 mmol Na$^+$); and 0.5–1.0 mmol/kg K$^+$ (40–70 mmol K$^+$).

When no expected oral intake (ØGCS, unsafe swallow, post-CVA, preoperative, etc.), this may be provided as follows.

This '1 sour (0.9% saline), 2 sweet (5% glucose)' regimen may be used in fit preoperative patients. Otherwise, if there are abnormal losses such as fever, vomiting, diarrhoea etc., use normal (0.9%) saline unless liver failure (discussed hereunder) or if Na$^+$ outside normal range (Ø or ≠).

Date	Infusion Fluid	Volume	Additives If Any Drug and Dose	Rate of Admin	Dura -tion	Dr's Signature	Time Start- ed	Time Com- pleted	Set Up by Sig- nature	Batch No.
08/01	5% Glucose	1 litre	20 mmol KCl		8h	TN				
08/01	Normal saline	1 litre			8h	TN				
08/01	5% Glucose	1 litre	20 mmol KCl		8h	TN				

Figure 3.2 Drug chart showing how to write up intravenous fluids.

Always get senior help if unsure, as incorrectly prescribed fluids can be as dangerous as any other incorrectly used drug (Figure 3.2). Individual fluid and electrolyte requirements may differ substantially according to:

- Body habitus, age, residual oral intake, if on multiple iv drugs (which are sometimes given with significant amounts of fluid).
- Insensible losses (normally about 1 L/d). ≠Skin losses if fever or burns. ≠Lung losses in hyperventilation or inhalation burns.
- GI losses (normally about 0.2 L/d). Any vomiting (≠Cl⁻ content) or diarrhoea (≠K⁺ content) must be taken into account as well as less obvious causes, e.g. ileus, fistulae.
- Fluid compartment shifts, esp vasodilation with distributive shock if sepsis/anaphylaxis.

K⁺ CONSIDERATIONS

Do not give at > 10 mmol/h iv unless K⁺ dangerously low, when it can be given quicker.

Postoperative surgical patients often need less K⁺ in 1st 24 h, as K⁺ is released by cell necrosis (proportional to extent of surgery).

HANDY HINTS

- Check the following before prescribing any iv fluid:
  - **Clinical markers of hydration:** Temperature, skin turgor, mucous membranes, JVP, peripheral oedema, pulmonary oedema (basal crackles). Easy to overlook, yet simple and useful signs!

- **Recent input and output:** If at all concerned, ask nurses to commence a strict fluid balance chart. Consider also starting a daily weight chart.
- **Recent U&Es, esp K⁺:** Can use VBG to get an urgent result, before lab bloods are available.

- In general, encourage oral fluids (often overlooked in the ED): homeostasis (if normal) is safer, less expensive and less consuming of doctor/nurse time than iv fluids. Beware of shock, fever, vomiting, diarrhoea or ileus (iv fluid will be needed); ↓swallow; fluid overload (esp if HF or RF); ↓GCS; or if homeostasis disorders (esp SIADH).
- Take extreme care if major organ failure:
    - **Heart failure:** Heart can quickly become 'overloaded' and ⇒ acute LVF. Even if not currently in HF, beware if predisposed (e.g. Hx of HF or IHD).
    - **Renal failure:** Unless pre-renal cause (e.g. hypovolaemia), do not give more fluid than residual renal function can deal with. Seek help from senior doctor if at all concerned; good fluid Mx greatly influences outcomes in this group. Use saline unless specialist advice taken.
    - **Liver failure:** Often preferable to use 5% glucose. Serum Na⁺ may be ↓d, but total body Na⁺ is often ↑d. Additional saline will end up in the wrong compartment (e.g. peritoneal fluid; therefore, ↑ing ascites) but may be essential to ensure renal perfusion (RF often coexists).
- If in doubt, give 'fluid challenges': small volumes (normally 200–500 mL) of fluid over short periods of time, to see whether clinical response to BP, urine output or left ventricular function is beneficial or detrimental before committing to longer-term fluid strategy.

HANDY HINTS
It can be difficult to elicit all this information under time pressure. The trick is to know when to take extreme care. Be particularly careful if you do not know the patient, i.e. a handover, and be wary when asked to 'just write up another bag' without reviewing

the patient. You may be asked to prescribe fluids when no longer necessary or even when they may be harmful. To save time for those on ward call (and to ≠ the chances of your patient getting appropriate fluids), leave clear instructions with the nurses and on the drug chart for as long as can be sensibly predicted (esp over weekends/long holidays).

Check the following before prescribing any iv fluid:

1. **Clinical markers of hydration:** temperature, skin turgor, mucous membranes, JVP, peripheral oedema, pulmonary oedema (basal crackles). Easy to overlook, yet simple and useful signs!
2. **Recent input and output:** if ANY at all concerned, ask nurses to commence a strict fluid balance chart. Consider also starting a daily weight chart.
3. **Recent U&Es, esp K$^+$.** Can use VBG to get an urgent result, before lab bloods are available.

- In general, encourage oral fluids (often overlooked in the ED): homeostasis (if normal) is safer, less expensive and less consuming of doctor/nurse time than iv fluids. Beware of shock, fever, vomiting, diarrhoea or ileus (iv fluid will be needed); ↓swallow; fluid overload (esp if HF or RF); ↓GCS; or if homeostasis disorders (esp SIADH).
- Take extreme care if major organ failure:

1. **Heart failure:** heart can quickly become 'overloaded' and ⇒ acute LVF. Even if not currently in HF, beware if predisposed (e.g. Hx of HF or IHD).
2. **Renal failure:** unless pre-renal cause (e.g. hypovolaemia), do not give more fluid than residual renal function can deal with. Seek help from senior doctor if at all concerned; good fluid Mx greatly influences outcomes in this group. Use saline unless specialist advice taken.
3. **Liver failure:** often preferable to use 5% glucose. Serum Na$^+$ may be ↓d, but total body Na$^+$ is often ↑d. Additional saline will end up in the wrong compartment (e.g. peritoneal fluid

∴ ↑ing ascites) but may be essential to ensure renal perfusion (RF often coexists).

4. **ARDS/ALI:** Can make fluid Rx difficult due to non-cardiogenic pulmonary oedema. Additionally, patients are often shocked with multi-organ failure. No consensus over exact fluid regimen, but preferable to adopt a 'dry' approach wherever possible by limiting fluid management to plasma expanders and closely monitoring urine output (support with inotropes if required).

- If in doubt, give 'fluid challenges': small volumes (normally 200–500 mL) of fluid over short periods of time, to see whether clinical response to BP, urine output or left ventricular function is beneficial or detrimental before committing to longer-term fluid strategy.

OXYGEN

ACUTE OXYGEN DELIVERY

Oxygen (O_2) is an important Rx for many acute respiratory and non-respiratory diseases. It is most commonly used acutely when $SaO_2 < 92\%$ ($PaO_2 < 8$ kPa). Delivery can be either **'controlled'** or **'uncontrolled'** (Box 3.5.1).

3.5.1 Controlled or uncontrolled O_2 therapy?

Uncontrolled O_2 is suitable for most situations.
Controlled O_2 should be considered when extra O_2 is required, but ventilation is heavily dependent on hypoxic drive rather than CO_2 chemoreceptors, e.g. chronic ↑PCO_2 associated with neuromuscular weakness, chest wall deformity, obesity or exacerbations of COPD and CF. Targeted O_2 saturation should be 88–92%. Patient O_2 alert cards are helpful.

Uncontrolled oxygen

Achieved with a number of different devices:

1. *Nasal cannulae* ('prongs') set to a specific flow rate (usually 1–5 L/min) and titrated to SaO_2. Paediatric flowmeters can also be used to achieve flows < 1 L/min, e.g. in COPD. Prongs are more comfortable and allow eating and drinking; however, O_2 delivery is unpredictable.
2. *High-flow face masks* ('Hudson mask') can deliver ↑ O_2 concentrations (50–60%) and are controlled by regulating the flow rate (usually > 5 L/min).
3. *Non-rebreathe masks* are used when high-flow face masks cannot achieve SaO_2 > 92%. They have a reservoir at their base which contains 100% O_2 and is protected from exhaled CO_2 by a one-way valve. They deliver between 60% and 80% FiO_2 (10–15 L/min).

Controlled oxygen

Achieved via a *Venturi mask*. O_2 can be carefully titrated during CO_2 retention (target SaO_2 = 88–92%). Venturi mask works by setting the O_2 flow to the rate written on the nozzle. O_2 is directed through the narrow nozzle, which lowers the pressure to draw in surrounding air. The amount of air that mixes with the O_2 determines the O_2 concentration delivered to the patient.
Available: Blue (2 L/min = 24%), white (4 L/min = 28%), orange (6 L/min = 31%), yellow (8 L/min = 35%), red (10 L/min = 40%) and green (12 L/min = 60%).

High-flow oxygen therapy via nasal cannula (Optiflow™ Airvo™)

Newer systems which deliver high-flow rates of humidified oxygen (up to 50 L/min) through specialised nasal cannulae. Increasingly used for type 1 respiratory failure. Work by 'washing out' the anatomical dead space and exerting a low level of PEEP to enable alveolar recruitment.

DOMICILIARY (HOME) OXYGEN THERAPY

Different prescriptions are possible and patients may be prescribed more than one: (1) **Long-term O_2 therapy** (LTOT; Rx of chronic hypoxia, most commonly COPD); (2) **Ambulatory O_2** (AOT; to allow greater activity by relieving associated SOB); (3) **Short burst O_2 therapy** (SBOT; for relief of SOB, e.g. after exertion; now rarely justified); (4) **Nocturnal O_2 therapy** (NOT; to correct nocturnal hypoxaemia); (5) **Palliative O_2 therapy** (POT; to relieve sensation of SOB with terminal conditions).

- **LTOT:** Indicated for many conditions with chronic $PaO_2 \leq 7.3$ kPa (or 55 mmHg) *or* PaO_2 7.3–8 kPa (or 55–60 mmHg) with 2° polycythaemia, peripheral oedema or pulmonary hypertension (Box 3.5.2). Prescribed for ≥ 15 h/d (to include the night) with aim to $\uparrow PaO_2 > 8$ kPa (or 60 mmHg). An initial prescription might be 1 L/min. **Assessment:** (1) check resting O_2 sats $\leq 92\%$ (or $\leq 94\%$ if polycythaemia, peripheral oedema or pulmonary hypertension); (2) ensure patient is stable (> 8 wks after exacerbation); (3) ensure on optimal Rx; (4) ideally ensure $2 \times$ ABGs > 3 wks apart meet above criteria; (5) ABG also taken > 30 min on O_2 to ensure $PaO_2 > 8$ kPa (and to assess CO_2). **NB:** some centres use a combination of pulse oximetry, capillary blood gas sampling (CBG) and cutaneous capnography to perform LTOT assessments. ☠ CO_2 retention

---

3.5.2 Indications for LTOT

- COPD
- Severe chronic asthma
- ILD
- CF
- Bronchiectasis
- Pulmonary vascular disease
- Primary pulmonary hypertension
- Pulmonary malignancy
- Nocturnal hypoventilation, usually with NIV or CPAP (e.g. obesity, neuromuscular or restrictive lung disorders and OSA)

may not be evident on 30 min ABG but may occur overnight; therefore, warn patients of possible symptoms. ☠ Patients with a significant rise in $PaCO_2$ (> 1 kPa) on > 1 occasion should only be offered LTOT in conjunction with NIV.

- **AOT:** Supplemental O_2 to be used for exertion or activities of daily living. Can be prescribed on its own **OR** in combination with LTOT (usually required if LTOT patient is not housebound). Two-month assessment period is essential to adjust the prescription (both HR required/day AND rate in L/min, usually 3–6) AND to confirm clinical benefit (O_2 sats > 90% throughout exercise and objective improvement in exercise tolerance). Many different options available, e.g. conserver devices (delivery during inspiration only), portable concentrators, lightweight or self-filling cylinders and liquid O_2.
- **SBOT:** Used intermittently for short periods (e.g. 10–20 min) to relieve SOB not relieved by any other treatments. Traditionally prescribed for non-hypoxic patients to relieve 'subjective' SOB (e.g. during recovery from exertion). May also have a role in Rx of cluster headaches.
- **NOT:** O_2 administered overnight only. Nocturnal or sleep-related ↓PaO_2 can develop before daytime hypoxia is evident (worsening V/Q mismatch when supine ± lack of drive to ventilatory muscles). Nocturnal ↓PaO_2 may also be seen with cardiac failure. (inc. Cheyne–Stokes). Demonstrated on overnight oximetry. NB: always ensure LTOT ± nocturnal NIV is NOT more appropriate.
- **POT:** O_2 to relieve the sensation of refractory and persistent SOB associated with advanced or life-limiting disease (i.e. no relief with opiates). Best for those with resting O_2 sats < 92% **OR** those with normal O_2 sats who fail to respond to other Rx.

Important points to consider when prescribing home O_2:

1. Should *NOT* be prescribed to patients who smoke (fire hazard)
2. Comprehensive risk assessment should be completed before considering oxygen

3. LTOT is provided via an O_2 concentrator (0.5–8 L/min), but a backup cylinder should be available in case of power failure
4. Patients may adjust the flow rate for exercise or for sleep
5. Nasal prongs or controlled O_2 masks (Venturi) are available
6. The prescriber must complete a **Home Oxygen Order Form (HOOF)** and return by fax to the relevant supplier; **HOOF Part A** (non-specialists; for temporary provision of O_2) or **HOOF Part B** (specialist prescription after full assessment). **NB:** all information must be completed or the HOOF will be returned! The patient must also sign a consent form to allow disclosure of confidential information. Home O_2 is usually delivered in 3 days but a next day (or 4 h) service is available.
7. The Fire Service should be notified of patients who are using domiciliary O_2.

SEDATION FOR BRONCHOSCOPY

Bronchoscopy usually performed under sedation to provide anxiolysis and anterograde amnesia. Some operators may prefer not to sedate patients, esp under certain circumstances (e.g. elderly or patients with COPD). Ideal depth of sedation is 'conscious sedation', i.e. verbal contact is maintained at all times with airway patency and cardiorespiratory function intact.

 Important points to consider before administering sedation:

- Patients should always be fasted (ideally ≥ 6 h).
- Patients should be haemodynamically stable.
- Avoid sedation with respiratory compromise. **NB:** many patients with stable and non-severe chronic respiratory conditions may still be suitable but sedate with extra caution!
- Ensure adequate iv access.
- Ensure continual monitoring is attached to patient (O_2 saturations, HR).
- Administer O_2 (nasal O_2 is usual BUT high-flow O_2 should always be readily available!).

- Ensure easy access to antagonist drugs (e.g. flumazenil or naloxone); if reversal is required, use flumazenil to reverse the effects of midazolam first, except if a large opioid dose was administered. **NB:** half-life of antagonists < half-life of sedative → monitor for re-sedation.
- Start with small doses and assess response before titrating, in order to avoid over-sedation. **NB:** response to sedatives is highly variable!
- Continually assess level of sedation to ensure 'conscious sedation' and avoid over-sedation.

USUAL DRUG REGIMEN

Benzodiazepine (for sedation, anxiolysis, anterograde amnesia) ± an opioid (for analgesia, sedation and cough suppression). **NB:** if using an opioid, always administer it first and allow the full effect to be reached! **Typically regimen:** iv midazolam ± iv alfentanyl (doses discussed in Table 3.9).

Table 3.9 Common drugs used when sedating for bronchoscopy

Drug	Initial IV bolus	Subsequent dose	Typical effects	Antagonist
Midazolam	2 mg (0.5–1 mg in elderly)	0.5–1 mg (max. 10 mg)	Onset: 2 min Max. effect: 5–10 min Duration: 30 min–2 h	**Flumazenil** 200 mcg iv in 15 sec (+ further 100 mcg/min until response; max. 1 mg)
Alfentanyl	250 mcg	250 mcg (max. 500 mcg)	Onset: immediate Max. effect: immediate Duration: 30 min–1 h	**Naloxone** 200 mcg iv (+ further 100 mcg/2 min until response or consider infusion)
Fentanyl	25 mcg	25 mcg (max. 50 mcg)	Onset immediate Max. 5 min Duration 30 min–1 h	

Doses suggested are for guidance only; always consider your patient and seek advice if necessary.

Criteria for discharge and important points to consider:

- Alert and orientated (or returned to pre-procedure state)
- Ambulates safely (or returned to pre-procedure state)
- Discharged into care of responsible adult
- No driving or operating of machinery for 24 h
- Avoid alcohol or CNS depressant for 24 h

CORTICOSTEROIDS AND OTHER IMMUNOSUPPRESSIVE AGENTS

Corticosteroids and other immunosuppressive agents are used to Rx for many respiratory conditions. Centres differ in their use of many of these drugs → always consult local guidelines.

3.7.1 Some general advice

- ↑infection risk and more severe, atypical presentations, atypical organisms/TB reactivation.
- Avoid live vaccinations (e.g. measles, mumps, rubella, BCG, yellow fever, polio).
- Avoid exposure to varicella-zoster (shingles or chicken-pox) and measles (use Ig therapy if exposed).
- Prior to commencing AND during Rx always check the following:
  - **Azathioprine** → FBC, LFT & TPMT test. Recheck FBC at least every week for 2 month, then every 3 months. Recheck LFT monthly. Stop Rx if ↓WCC/Plt or ↑LFT.
  - **Corticosteroids** → BP, BM, consider osteopenia/osteoporosis (bisphosphonate).
  - **Cyclophosphamide** → FBC, U&E, LFT, Urine dipstick (haemorrhagic cystitis) and store semen. Recheck all every week for 1 month then every 2 months.
  - **Methotrexate** → FBC, U&E, LFT, CXR, folic acid. Recheck bloods before each dose (iv) or every week until at stable dose then monthly (po). Pregnancy test prior to commencing.

CORTICOSTEROIDS

Commonly used corticosteroids include:

Drug	Equivalent dose	Main respiratory uses
Prednisolone	5 mg	Acute exacerbations of asthma/COPD/ILD
Methylprednisolone	4 mg	Vasculitis, ILD
Dexamethasone	750 mcg	↑ICP or spinal metastasis
Hydrocortisone	20 mg	Acute asthma/COPD (iv)

Glucocorticoid fx predominate; mineralocorticoid fx for these are all mild apart from hydrocortisone (has moderate fx) and dexamethasone (has minimal fx, therefore, used when H_2O and Na^+ retention are particularly undesirable, e.g. ↑ICP).

Side effects = Cushing's syndrome!

Metabolic: Na^+/fluid retention*, hyperlipoproteinaemia, leukocytosis, negative K^+/Ca^{2+}/nitrogen balance, generalised fluid/electrolyte abnormalities.

Endocrine: Hyperglycaemia/↓GTT (can ⇒ DM), adrenal suppression.

Fat*: Truncal obesity, moon face, interscapular ('buffalo hump') and suprascapular fat pads.

Skin: Hirsutism, bruising/purpura, acne, striae, ↓healing, telangiectasia, thinning.

Other: Impotence, fx on foetus, menstrual irregularities/amenorrhoea, ↓growth (children), ↑appetite*.

GI: Pancreatitis, peptic/oesophageal ulcers: give PPI if on ↑doses.

Cardiac: HTN, CCF, myocardial rupture post-MI, TE.

Musculoskeletal: Proximal myopathy, osteoporosis, fractures (can ⇒ avascular necrosis).

Neurological: ↑epilepsy, ↑ICP/papilloedema (esp children on withdrawal of corticosteroids).

Ψ: Mood Δs (↑ or ↓), psychosis (esp at ↑doses), dependence.

Ocular: Cataracts, glaucoma, corneal/scleral thinning.

Infections: ↑susceptibility, ↑speed (↑severity at presentation), TB reactivation, ↑ risk PCP, ↑risk of chickenpox/shingles/measles. Avoid live vaccines if on long-term prednisolone > 20 mg.

3.7.2 SEs are dose-dependent

If patient is on high doses, make sure this is intentional: it is not rare in fluctuating (e.g. inflammatory) illnesses for patients to be left on high doses by mistake. Seek advice if unsure.
If on long-term Rx consider giving Ca^{2+}/vit D supplements/bisphosphonate to ↓risk of osteoporosis[1] and PPI to ↓risk of GI ulcer. Ensure hypertension and blood glucose are controlled. Ensure patient carries a steroid Rx card.

---

1 *To reduce risk of osteoporosis use lowest possible dose and shortest possible course. Current guidelinesRCP recommend: (1) DEXA scan for patients who will be on ≥ 7.5 mg prednisolone (or equivalent) for ≥ 3 months and bisphosphonates if ↓bone mineral density (T score ≤ – 1.5). (2) Start bisphosphonate if ≥ 1 other risk factor (e.g. age > 65 or previous osteoporotic fracture).*

3.7.3 Cautions

Can mostly be worked out from the SEs, e.g. if patient already has a condition that is a potential SE (e.g. DM). Systemic corticosteroids are CI in systemic infections (w/o antibiotic cover). **NB:** Avoid live vaccines. If never had chickenpox, avoid exposure.

Interactions
Apply to all systemic Rx. fx can be ↓d, e.g. by rifampicin, carbamazepine, phenytoin and phenobarbital, may need to increase dose (double dose if on rifampicin), fx can be ↑d, e.g. by erythromycin, ketoconazole, itraconazole and ciclosporin (whose own fx are ↑d by methylprednisolone). ↑risk of ↓K^+ with amphotericin and digoxin.

Withdrawal effects
Sudden withdrawal can precipitate acute adrenal insufficiency (= Addisonian crisis; ☠ can be fatal ☠): ↓BP (can be postural),

↑HR, weakness, fever, myalgia, arthralgia, abdominal pain, vomiting, rhinitis, conjunctivitis, painful itchy nodules, ↓Wt, confusion (and coma) and characteristic electrolyte changes (↓Na$^+$, ↑K$^+$, ↑Ur, ↑Cr, ↓CBG); therefore, must withdraw slowly if patient has had > 3 wks Rx (or a shorter course within 1 yr of stopping long-term Rx), other causes of adrenal suppression, received high doses (> 40 mg od prednisolone or equivalent) or repeat doses in evening, or repeat course. **NB:** intercurrent illness, trauma, surgery needs ↑doses and can precipitate relative withdrawal.

AZATHIOPRINE

Cytotoxic agent. Less effective than cyclophosphamide → used second line in Rx of pulmonary vasculitis (steroid-sparing). Also for ILD, sarcoid or to prevent transplant rejection. Takes ≈ 4 wks to work and maximal effect often not seen for months.

3.7.4 Thiopurine methyltransferase (TPMT)

TPMT metabolises thiopurine drugs (azathioprine, mercaptopurine, tioguanine): ↑risk of myelosuppression with ↓enzyme activity: 90% of population have normal TPMT activity, 10% have intermediate activity and ≈ 0.3% no activity.
   Always measure TPMT activity before starting azathioprine: patients with no TPMT activity should not receive thiopurine drugs; those with intermediate activity may be Rx but **ONLY** under close supervision (↓dose esp if taking aminosalicylate derivatives).

Dose: Start 1–3 mg/kg/daily po (☠ avoid iv as very irritant ☠). NB: ↓dose with RF or LF.

CYCLOPHOSPHAMIDE

Alkylating agent (cross-links DNA bases). Both cytotoxic and immunosuppressive → used for some cancers and is the 1° *cytotoxic drug for pulmonary vasculitis* (combined with corticosteroids ≈ 90%

remission). Also used occasionally for 'inflammatory lung fibrosis' associated with connective tissue disease. Often reserved for severe cases (life- or organ-threatening).

Dose

Rx can be po or via pulsed iv; similar remission rates, but iv often preferred as ↓ cumulative dose and; therefore, ↓side effects. **Always consult local hospital policy before prescribing!** The following is a guide *only*[SPC].

 Pulsed iv cyclophosphamide: 500 mg/m^2 (body surface area calculated using the DuBois formula: http://www.halls.md/body-surface-area/bsa.htm) at 3–4 wkly intervals. Always prescribe anti-emetics, **MESNA** (during and after infusion) and co-trimoxazole (see Box 3.7.5). Use adjusted body weight if BMI >30 (27.5 × height squared).

 Rx usually for 3–6 months *only* (six doses) depending on response and adverse effects (> 6 months ↑risk side effects). Typically 'induce remission' with cyclophosphamide + low-dose corticosteroid then 'maintain remission' with corticosteroid + 2° immunosuppressant (azathioprine or methotrexate) over longer term.

3.7.5 Cyclophosphamide considerations

- Takes ≈ 2 wks until effects are seen; therefore, combine with po corticosteroids (usually low dose < 10 mg prednisolone).
- Risk of haemorrhagic cystitis (from urinary metabolite acrolein) and bladder cancer; therefore,
  - Monitor urine dipstick for blood (several years if large cumulative dose).
- Prescribe sodium 2-mercaptoethanesulfonate (Mesna) as a regional chelator.
- Ensure good hydration (> 3L/24 h ± 1 L ivi n/saline pre iv dose).
- Store semen before starting Rx (males) and ensure negative pregnancy test (females).
- Ensure contraception: females of child bearing age should use contraception during and for 12 months post-Rx, males should use contraception during and for 6 months post-Rx.

- PCP prophylaxis with co-trimoxazole; usually 12 months.
- If ↓WCC stop po Rx or postpone next dose if iv. Allow WCC to recover and restart at ↓dose (≈ 25–50% reduction).

METHOTREXATE

An antimetabolite. **Dose:** start 7.5–10 mg po once/wk (↑according to disease and haematological response by 2.5 mg wkly, max. 25 mg). Prescriber should specify day of intake on the prescription.

3.7.6 Methotrexate considerations

- **Dose is weekly!** (☠ daily administration can be lethal ☠)
- Toxic to lung (chronic toxicity more common than acute)
  - Baseline CXR before starting Rx
  - Stop if any Sx or signs suggesting fibrosis/pneumonitis
- Can accumulate in pleural effusions and ascites → highly toxic if returns to circulation
  - Drain effusions or ascites before starting Rx
- Prescribe with folic acid 5 mg po od (omitted on day of methotrexate and day after)
- Ensure adequate contraception during treatment

MYCOPHENOLATE MOFETIL (CELLCEPT)

Suppression of lymphocyte numbers and function. Often used po as immunosuppressant in ILD, esp ILD associated with connective tissue disease. **Dose:** typically 1–1.5 g bd po (start 250–500 mg po bd and uptitrate in 250 mg bd increments 2–4 wkly while monitoring FBC) but follow local guidance. **VITAL:** always prescribe as mycophenolate mofetil (mycophenolate sodium is different dose). ☠ Beware infection (withhold) and closely monitor FBC as leucopenia, thrombocytopenia, anaemia, pancytopenia and leucocytosis are all commonly reported ☠. **NB:** mycophenolate (and its metabolites) are associated with a high rate of birth defects and spontaneous abortion; pregnancy tests should be performed before commencing (two negative tests 8–10 days apart^{MHRA}) and patients should be counselled on the use of effective contraception during Rx and for up to 3 months after.

THROMBOLYSIS

Fibrinolytic drugs, which activate plasminogen → plasmin → fibrin degradation. Indicated for Rx of 'massive' PE and considered for 'submassive' PE (controversial; risk *vs.* benefit less clear).

3.8.1 Contraindications to thrombolysis (PE)

NB: No contraindications are absolute in patients with suspected large PE who have arrested (or peri-arrest). Contraindications are important to consider prior to thrombolysis for 'submassive' PE:

Absolute:

- Intracranial haemorrhage or stroke of unknown origin at any time
- Ischaemic stroke in preceding 6 months
- CNS damage, atrioventricular malformation or neoplasms
- Major trauma/surgery/head injury < 3 wks
- GI bleeding < 1 month
- Known bleeding disorder (excluding menses)
- Aortic dissection
- Non-compressible punctures in last 24 h (e.g. liver biopsy, lumbar puncture)

Relative:

- TIA < 6 months
- Oral anticoagulant therapy
- Pregnancy or < 1 wk postpartum
- Prolonged or traumatic resuscitation
- Refractory hypertension (systolic > 180 mmHg and/or diastolic > 110 mmHg)
- Advanced liver disease

Also commonly used for acute MI (although primary angioplasty now more common), ischaemic stroke, arterial (or venous) TE, e.g. DVT, central retinal venous (or arterial) thrombosis or for clearing clotted catheters/cannulas. Most fibrinolytics are only licensed for some of these indications[BNF]. Always consider contraindications (discussed hereunder) before deciding to thrombolyse PE. There may be no choice with 'massive' PE (Rx life-saving!) (Box 3.8.1).

Common side effects are bleeding (mostly mild and at iv sites; if severe or suspect cerebral bleed occurring, stop ivi and get senior help!), N&V, ↓BP (transient and often improves if ↓rate of ivi and raise legs). Mild hypersensitivity (inc uveitis) can also occur. Anaphylaxis and GBS occur rarely.

ADMINISTRATION OF THROMBOLYSIS FOR PE

Alteplase (recombinant tissue type plasminogen activator (rt-PA); ACTILYSE) is the agent of choice, but other agents can be used in an emergency when alteplase is not available. Always use your hospital's protocol if one exists! – contact HDU, ITU, CCU, A&E or look on your hospital Intranet for details. Doses depend on the indication for thrombolysis. The following is a suggested approach for PE:

1. Administer alteplase (total dose: 100 mg if > 65 kg or 1.5 mg/kg if < 65 kg)
   - Initial 10 mg iv bolus (1–2 min)
   - Administer remainder of dose as ivi over 2 h (e.g. 90 mg for patient > 65 kg)
   - In cardiac arrest or massive PE with imminent cardiac arrest → 50 mg as iv bolus can be given

2. After thrombolysis start UFH (**NB:** different to standard UFH regimens):
   - iv bolus – 60 units/kg (max. 4000 units)
   - ivi at 12 units/kg/h (max. 1000 units/h) and adjust rate to maintain APTT 50–70 sec
   - Continue for 24–48 h (then can convert to LMWH)

Alteplase should be administered in monitored setting, normally A&E resus, CCU, HDU or ITU. Patients should remain on bed rest for 24–48 h. Observations should be regular: e.g. every 15 min for 2 h, every 30 min for 6 h, then hrly. ☠ If intracranial haemorrhage occurs, consider 5–10 units cryoprecipitate (± platelets ± FFP) and seek early neurosurgical opinion ☠.

If thrombolysis for submassive PE is contraindicated or high risk of bleeding: consider referral for embolectomy, half-dose thrombolysis (↓risk) or catheter-directed thrombolysis.

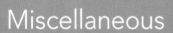

Miscellaneous

DOI: 10.1201/9781315151816-4

CHEST DRAINS AND PLEURAL PROCEDURES

CHEST DRAINS

☠ The National Patient Safety Agency (NPSA) issued a rapid response report (2008) which highlighted the dangers of chest drain insertion: http://www.nrls.npsa.nhs.uk/resources/?entryid45=59887; it can result in significant complications, including death ☠. ALWAYS carefully consider whether a chest drain is required or whether an alternative safer procedure (e.g. aspiration) could be performed (Box 4.1.1). If the case is complex or if any doubt, consult respiratory team. ☠. USS guidance is required for all drains inserted for fluid (but not for pneumothorax) ☠. ALWAYS consult the BTS website for the latest guidance: https://www.brit-thoracic.org.uk/guidelines-and-quality-standards.

4.1.1 Chest drain indications and contraindications

Indications:
- Pneumothorax, including tension
- Parapneumonic effusion or empyema
- Malignant pleural effusion for symptomatic relief and pleurodesis
- Haemothorax/haemopneumothorax
- Post-thoracic surgery (ALWAYS consult cardiothoracic surgeons first)
- Symptomatic relief for effusions of any other aetiology (consider therapeutic aspiration instead!)

Contraindications:
- Inexperienced operator
- Lung known to be adherent to lung wall ($\rightarrow$ failure to reinflate and relieve Sx)
- INR > 1.5, ↓↓platelets or bleeding tendency (relative contraindication; correct if possible)
- Post-pneumonectomy (relative contraindication; discuss with cardiothoracics first)

Guide to chest drain insertion

Prior to insertion:

1. Confirm indication (e.g. review patient and CXR) and ensure no contraindications
2. Discuss procedure with patient and obtain written consent
3. Ensure an assistant is present and a procedure room available
4. Ensure IV cannula inserted
5. Select preferred chest drain type; *Seldinger drain* (usually more comfortable to insert) or *blunt dissection drain*
6. Select drain size: *smaller drains* (10–14 F) are more comfortable and easy to insert when the intercostal space is narrow, while *larger drains* (>18 F) are often uncomfortable but may be preferred with larger air leaks, surgical emphysema, haemothorax or highly purulent empyema
7. Offer patient pre-procedure analgesia (e.g. **oramorph 10 mg** ≈ 15 min before commencing). **NB:** sedation is rarely required

Stepwise approach to insertion:

1. **Position of patient:** either sat at 45° in bed with arm held behind head (most often for pneumothorax) or with patient sitting forward leaning over a table (most often for effusion).
2. **Choose insertion site:** within 'safe triangle' (discussed hereunder) for pneumothorax or located with USS for effusions (either 'real-time' or by marking the site immediately before starting). ☠ Avoid posterior approaches close to the midline as intercostal arteries run more medially in this position ☠ (Figure 4.1).
3. Sterilise the skin and wear sterile gloves and gown.
4. Anaesthetise the skin, intercostal muscles and parietal pleura with adequate 1% lignocaine, usually 10–20 mL (max. dose 3 mg/kg) using a green needle. Aim just above the upper border of the rib (avoids neurovascular bundle) and verify the correct site by aspirating fluid or air (green needle may be too short for obese patients). **NB:** you can use this step as a guide for the depth of the pleural space relative to the skin surface.
5. Allow time for the local anaesthetic to take effect (can prepare rest of drainage equipment during this time).

6. Insert the drain:
   - **Seldinger technique:** Insert introducer needle and pull back on syringe until air or fluid is aspirated. Remove the syringe and pass the guidewire through the introducer needle. ☠ Never let go of the guidewire! ☠ Remove the introducer needle and make a small incision at the entry-point of the wire to allow easy passage of the dilator to create a tract. ☠ Never insert the dilator too far or with too much force! ☠ Remove the dilator and slide the drain along the wire. Remove the wire.
   - **Blunt dissection technique:** Make a small incision parallel to the rib. Carefully dissect through the tissue planes with a blunt forceps (opening and closing) ± finger. This can take some time. Once dissected, introduce the drain using the plastic introducer or loaded onto the forceps. ☠ Never introduce using the trocar. ☠
7. Connect the drain to an underwater seal (bottle filled with water to the line) via a three-way tap.
8. Ensure the drain is swinging with respiration and bubbling (pneumothorax) or draining fluid (effusion).
9. Suture the drain in position and secure to the chest wall (usually with tape/dressing).
10. Offer the patient further analgesia (+ prescribe PRN on drug chart).
11. Warn the patient not to disconnect the tube or any tubing, lift the bottle above chest height, or kink the tube (most commonly by lying on it).
12. Order CXR to confirm correct position. Effective drainage does not require an apical (pneumothorax) or basal position (effusion). Do NOT reposition or reinsert for this reason.
13. Consider prescribing regular flushes (10–20 mL normal saline), esp for very purulent effusions to avoid blockage.

Complications:

1. Pain (can be avoided with adequate local anaesthetic and *peri*-procedure analgesia)

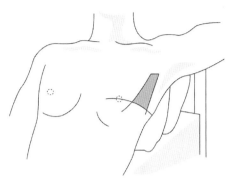

Figure 4.1 'Safe triangle' for chest drain insertion. It avoids major blood vessels and muscles. Bordered anteriorly by the border of pectoralis major, posteriorly by the border of latissimus dorsi, inferiorly by the level of the nipple or 5th intercostal space and superiorly by the base of the axilla.

2. Infection (intrapleural, wound or cellulitis)
3. Haemorrhage (if significant → immediately clamp drain, arrange urgent CT and discuss with cardiothoracics)
4. Surgical emphysema – Air leaking from a pneumothorax into subcutaneous tissues
5. Organ damage (e.g. lung, heart, great vessels, stomach, liver and spleen) – Continuous significant bubbling should raise the suspicion of an intrapulmonary insertion
6. Seeding of tumour along tract
7. Re-expansion pulmonary oedema
8. Vasovagal reaction
9. Death

Top Tips for drain management

1. Manage patients on specialist wards wherever possible
2. Ensure a drain is regularly checked and a chart completed

3. If a drain stops swinging consider whether it is kinked (often at skin under dressing), blocked (try gentle flushing), clamped or has come out (examine patient, drain site ± CXR).
4. High volume/low-pressure suction (5–20 cm H_2O) can be used to encourage drainage, esp for persisting air leaks.
5. Never clamp a bubbling chest drain (risk of tension pneumothorax)
6. Clamping can be considered for:
   a. Controlling the drainage of a large pleural effusion, where rapid drainage ↑risk of re-expansion pulmonary oedema.
   b. Detect on-going small air leaks, prior to deciding on removing a chest drain in an 'apparently' resolved pneumothorax. Clamping a chest drain for several hours and repeating a CXR can detect very slow or intermittent air leaks. However, always perform with caution on a specialist ward only, with regular observation and immediately unclamp the drain if the patient experiences any symptoms suggesting pneumothorax recurrence.

Removing chest drains
Opinions differ on whether drains should be removed with timed expiration or at maximal inspiration. Either way, remove drain quickly and smoothly, placing a suture to close the wound. CXR is required to ensure no post-removal pneumothorax.

Indwelling pleural catheters
Used in appropriate patients for the domiciliary drainage of recurring malignant pleural effusions. They are fenestrated silicone drains (softer) which tunnel subcutaneously for a short distance before entering the chest and pleural cavity. They should only be inserted by trained individuals after considering alternatives (e.g. standard drainage and pleurodesis). The patient drains independently by connecting a 'vacuumed' drainage bottle (1 L) to the valve at the end of the drain, usually performed 1–3 times/wk.

PLEURAL ASPIRATION

Otherwise known as a 'thoracentesis' or 'pleural tap'. A small volume of pleural fluid can be aspirated to help identify the cause of the effusion (**diagnostic aspiration**) or larger volumes can be aspirated from more extensive effusions to help relieve symptoms (**therapeutic aspiration**). ☠ As with chest drain insertion, USS should always be used to help guide aspiration of effusions ☠. Pneumothoraces can also be therapeutically aspirated[BTS] (page 267). There are no absolute contraindications, although ideally INR < 1.5. **Complications include:** pain, pneumothorax, cough, bleeding, infection (including empyema), organ puncture and malignant seeding.

Stepwise approach to diagnostic pleural aspiration (effusion):

1. Follow steps 1–5 of chest drain insertion (identical)
2. Aspirate using a 50-mL syringe and green needle (21 G)
3. Advance the needle while pulling back on syringe until fluid is aspirated
4. Note and record the appearance of the fluid (e.g. haemorrhagic or purulent)
5. Send appropriate samples (discussed hereunder)
6. Arrange CXR to exclude pneumothorax (or other complications) if: the patient is unwell, unable to aspirate fluid, very haemorrhagic or the procedure was difficult. A routine CXR is not normally recommended

Stepwise approach to therapeutic pleural aspiration (effusion and pneumothorax):

1. Follow steps 1–5 of chest drain insertion (identical)
2. Either use a green iv cannula, three-way tap and 50-mL syringe (± tubing and sterile jug for effusions) OR a commercially available pack (same contents but sealed sterile bag replaces the jug)
3. Advance the cannula while aspirating with the syringe
4. Once fluid or air is aspirated, remove the needle leaving the plastic cannula in situ (place a finger or cap over the end!)

5. Attach the three-way tap to the cannula. If aspirating for effusion, also attach the plastic tubing to the second port of the three-way tap, placing the other end inside the plastic jug. On the third port of the three-way tap attach the syringe

6. Using the syringe, aspirate pleural fluid from the pleural space, before turning the three-way tap and re-directing the fluid down the tubing and into the jug. For pneumothoraces, the additional tubing is not required

7. Aspirate a maximum of 1.5 L (risk of re-expansion pulmonary oedema). Always stop if resistance is felt or if pain/controllable coughing

8. USS is useful in demonstrating a reduction in pleural fluid

9. Send appropriate samples (discussed hereunder)

4.1.2 Pleural fluid – What to send

ALWAYS note and document the pleural fluid appearance (e.g. bloody, turbid, milky or pus)

Routine analysis:
   Biochemistry (can be sent in blood vacutainers) – Protein, glucose and LDH
   pH – Use heparinised ABG syringe and analyser (not if clearly purulent!); pH < 7.2 suggests empyema
   Cytology and **differential cell count** (send > 20 mL to ↑ yield of malignant cells)
   MC&S (including Gram stain)
   AFB and **TB culture** (↓ yield – may need to combine with histology)

Other tests:
If clinically indicated: cholesterol, triglycerides or chylomicrons (chylothorax), haematocrit (haemothorax), adenosine deaminase (TB) and amylase (pancreatitis).

PLEURAL BIOPSY

Pleural biopsy is occasionally required to help identify the aetiology of a pleural effusion. Best with either **image-guided pleural biopsy**

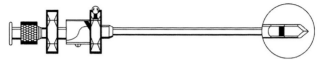

Figure 4.2 Abrams needle. Consists of two concentric tubes. The outer tube has a trocar point with a notch/window, which can be opened or closed by rotating the inner tube. A syringe can be loaded onto the end of the needle for aspiration.

(**usually CT**), which uses a cutting needle to core sections of parietal pleura *or* by biopsying **under direct vision at thoracoscopy/VATS**. These two methods are preferred[BTS]. However, multiple percutaneous pleural biopsies can also be obtained 'blindly' using an **'Abrams' needle** (Figure 4.2); poorer yield (≈ 50%) as pleural malignancy can be patchy. Now very rarely used in the diagnosis of malignant pleural disease. Most helpful with TB pleural disease. ☠ USS should always be used to help guide biopsy site. ☠ **Complications include:** pain, pneumothorax, haemothorax, infection (inc empyema) and intercostal artery injury (may require urgent cardiothoracic surgery).

Stepwise approach to Abrams needle pleural biopsy:

1. Perform with patient sat on edge of bed, leaning onto a table with their arms folded in front of them. A pillow can be used for comfort
2. Use US to identify best site: adequate depth of pleural fluid (to prevent inadvertent lung injury) ± targeting diseased pleura (e.g. visualised thickening or nodules)
3. Avoid posterior approaches, which can injury the neurovascular bundle
4. Follow steps 1–5 of chest drain insertion
5. Assemble Abrams needle
6. Make a small incision and bluntly dissect the intercostal muscles
7. Gently pass the needle with the window closed and facing downwards (6 o'clock). Confirm correct position by aspirating fluid using a syringe attached to the needle

8. Take a biopsy by angling the needle downwards and opening the window. Pull the window against the parietal pleura on the rib below by gently retracting the needle (a tug might be felt). Close the biopsy window to catch a sample of pleura. Remove the needle
9. Remove the sample from the window (can use a green needle)
10. Repeat step 8, sampling several times (≈ 5); always between 4 and 8 o'clock to avoid the neurovascular bundle
11. Suture the wound if necessary and apply a dressing
12. Send appropriate samples (e.g. in saline for TB and formalin for histology)
13. Always request CXR to exclude pneumothorax

FLYING AND DIVING

FLYING

Aircraft cabins are pressurised but flying can still cause a number of problems: $\downarrow PaO_2$, $\uparrow$volume of trapped gases (e.g. pneumothorax), transmission of infectious disease (e.g. TB), venous thromboembolism or exacerbations of symptoms (e.g. asthma or COPD).

☠The following are CONTRAINDICATIONS to flying: infectious TB, pneumothorax with persisting air leak, major haemoptysis, LTOT with a requirement > 4 L/min at sea level[BTS]☠.

Patients with the following conditions should undergo a pre-flight assessment (min. history and examination)[BTS]: severe COPD (FEV_1 < 30% predicted) or asthma, bullous lung disease, severe restrictive lung disease (VC < 1 L, esp with $\downarrow PaO_2$/$\uparrow PCO_2$), CF, comorbidity that could be worsened by $\downarrow PaO_2$ (e.g. CVD, IHD or pulmonary hypertension), pulmonary TB, < 6 wks following hospital discharge for acute respiratory illness, recent PTX, at risk of VTE, pre-existing requirement for O_2, CPAP/BiPAP (Box 4.2.1).

Hypoxia

Commercial aircraft cabins are pressurised to the minimum allowed altitude of 8000 ft (≈ 2400 m). At sea level $FiO_2 = 21$ kPa;

however, at 8000 ft $FiO_2 \approx 16$ kPa, which is the equivalent of breathing 15% O_2. Even in healthy subjects, this can result in a $PaO_2 \approx 8$ kPa (or sats $\approx 88–92\%$). Patients with significant lung disease are closer to the steep part of the Hb dissociation curve $\rightarrow$ proportionally greater $\downarrow$ Hb saturation at altitude. These patients should be considered for in-flight O_2 (discussed hereunder).

Logistics of in-flight O_2: Patients already on LTOT can travel with their own small cylinders or increasingly their lightweight battery-operated portable O_2 concentrators. However, the airline must be notified in advance! Patients NOT on O_2 at sea level, but those who require in-flight O_2 are prescribed either 2 L/min or 4 L/min via nasal cannulae, often using breath-activated pulsed systems. This is usually supplied by the airline, which will issue a MEDIF form to be completed by the patient and GP/specialist and returned for evaluation. **NB:** the need for O_2 on the ground (e.g. for connections or high altitude airports) must be organised separately by the patient.

4.2.1 Deciding whether O_2 should be prescribed for flying

Different centres use different methods to help make decisions. However, there is limited evidence to support for these methods. Always consult latest BTS guidance:

- https://www.brit-thoracic.org.uk/guidelines-and-quality-standards/air-travel-recommendations/

    Hypoxic challenge testing: Cabin altitudes (8000 ft) are crudely 'simulated' by breathing a nitrogen gas mixture ($\approx 15\%$ O_2) for 15–20 min. Sats and ABGs are performed $\rightarrow$ in-flight O_2 is prescribed if $PaO_2 < 6.6$ kPa *or* sats < 85%

    O_2 saturations and walk test (e.g. 6 min walk test): No universally agreed criteria. The following are suggested:

- Resting sats > 92% $\rightarrow$ no O_2 required
- Resting sats 90–92% $\rightarrow$ perform 6MWT and prescribe in-flight O_2 if sats < 85%
- Sats < 90% $\rightarrow$ prescribe in-flight O_2

> **Equations:** Several exist to help estimate PaO$_2$ at altitude.
> *Example:* PaO$_2$ at 8000 ft = (0.24 × PaO$_2$ sea level) + (2.7 ×
> FEV$_1$/FVC ratio) + 3; e.g. (0.24 × 8.2 kPa) + (2.7 × 0.5 ratio)
> + 3 = 6.3 kPa (in-flight O$_2$ recommended)

Pneumothorax

Ascent to 8000 ft increases volume of gas trapped in compartments
by ≈ 40%. ☠ Patients with a persisting pneumothorax should NOT
fly; those with a resolved pneumothorax (confirmed radiologically)
can only fly after 1 wk (2 wks if caused by trauma)[BTS] ☠. Patients fully
recovered from thoracic surgery can fly (previously advised 2 wks)[BTS].

Mycobacterium TB

☠ Patients with infectious TB should NOT travel by commercial
flight until their sputum is smear negative on at least two
occasions[WHO] or they have completed 2 wks of *effective*
treatment[BTS] ☠. **NB:** two smear negative sputum samples should
always be obtained with any cases of suspected or proven MDR-TB
or XDR-TB.

Venous thromboembolism

Current evidence is unclear and guidelines contradictory. Case-
by-case consideration required! Patients considered ↑ risk of VTE
should sit in an aisle seat, avoid excess alcohol/caffeine, remain
mobile and consider compression stockings. Those at ↑↑ risk
(e.g. past idiopathic VTE, < 6 wks after major trauma/surgery
or cancer) should be considered for temporary LMWH or formal
anticoagulation. ☠ Patients with VTE should NOT travel for 4 wks
or until DVT Sx have resolved ☠.

Exacerbations (Asthma or COPD)

In the event of exacerbation, patients can use their own
bronchodilator ± spacer. This can be as effective as a nebuliser.
Many airlines permit the use of dry cell battery-operated nebulisers:
this should be confirmed in advance. Patients can carry rescue
medication[NICE] (antibiotic + prednisolone). Regulations stipulate
that aircraft carry a bronchodilator inhaler in their emergency kit.

Other considerations

Lung cancer: Always consider the following pre-flight: correcting anaemia by transfusion, adequately draining pleural effusions, medical insurance and a doctor's letter for controlled drugs. ☠ Patients with SVCO, lymphangitis carcinomatosa, major haemoptysis or following a recent seizure (e.g. cerebral metastasis) should NOT fly ☠.

OSA: A doctor's letter is required outlining the diagnosis and requirement for CPAP. The machine must be dry cell battery operated and should be suitable for altitude and compatible with the power supply at the destination.

DIVING

Many chronic lung conditions are considered CONTRAINDICA-TIONS to diving (e.g. COPD, CF, ILD and lung bullae). Specific guidance for asthma and PTx is provided by the **British Sub-Aqua Club (BSAC):** http://www.bsac.com.

4.2.2 Diving and pneumothorax (BSAC)

Patients with spontaneous PTX MAY dive after:
- Definitive bilateral thoracic surgery
- 5 years have elapsed without any recurrence; provided a CT and lung function tests (inc flow-volume loops) suggest no residual lung disease

DIVING AND ASTHMA (BSAC)

The onset of acute asthma can be provoked by the dry gas inhaled from SCUBA apparatus. Uncontrolled asthma may also predispose to air trapping → lung barotrauma and air embolism. A preventive dose ß₂-agonist can be taken before a dive. ☠ Asthmatics must NOT dive if: ☠

- Poorly controlled (symptomatic, > occasional bronchodilator use, required therapeutic bronchodilator or PEFR > 15% below best value within 48 h of dive)
- Cold-, exercise- or emotion-induced asthma

Barotrauma

During descent and ascent, there are changes to the pressure exerted on air-filled cavities (inc lungs) → forces air out of and into the cavity respectively. Pulmonary barotrauma is most frequently caused by breath-holding during ascent: compressed gas in lung expands as external pressure falls → lung overexpansion and rupture. Can result in PTX (tension), pneumomediastinum and air emboli. Rx = high flow or hyperbaric O_2.

The bends

Nitrogen dissolves into the blood and tissue fluids under high pressure. During ascent, this nitrogen bubbles off. If ↑amount bubbling off (e.g. during a rapid ascent), it can act as emboli → micro-infarction, clotting and inflammation within multiple organs. Reduced by: limiting diving times, slow ascent and breathing mixtures containing helium rather than nitrogen. Rx = hyperbaric O_2.

NON-INVASIVE AND CONTINUOUS POSITIVE AIRWAY PRESSURE VENTILATION

Ventilators can be **invasive** (via ETT/tracheostomy) or **non-invasive** (via face/nasal masks). Here, we consider **non-invasive ventilation (NIV) ONLY**. It is a form of positive pressure ventilation, i.e. ventilation is supported by the positive pressure delivered by a ventilator (**Remember:** unassisted ventilation arises from the negative pressure generated by chest expansion). It is also known as bi-level ventilation or BiPAP. Negative pressure ventilators are also available. They 'suck out' the chest wall during inspiration but are now rarely used and only for chronic respiratory failure (e.g. the iron lung or 'cuirasse' ventilator). **Continuous positive airway pressure (CPAP)** is not strictly a form of 'ventilation' but is also considered here.

4.3.1 Mechanical ventilation, NIV or CPAP for acute respiratory failure?

Decision-making can be difficult! Always involve a senior clinician ± ITU. 💀 DO NOT delay invasive ventilation for suitable patients by instigating NIV or CPAP 💀.

NIV/CPAP is most appropriate for unsuitable ITU candidates and the immunocompromised (e.g. AIDS and PCP). Broadly-speaking, if a non-invasive approach is taken, then:

- Type 1 Respiratory Failure → CPAP or High-flow Nasal Cannuale (e.g. Optiflow™ Airvo™)
- Type 2 (hypercapnic) Respiratory Failure → NIV

NON-INVASIVE VENTILATION (NIV; AKA BI-LEVEL VENTILATION OR BIPAP)

Pressure (± supplemental FiO_2) is delivered with respiration. There are two adjustable pressure settings (hence 'bi-level or -PAP): a pressure for expiration (expiratory positive airway pressure; **EPAP**) and a higher pressure during inspiration (inspiratory positive airway pressure; **IPAP**). The difference between the IPAP and EPAP is called the **pressure support** (**PS**). PS determines ventilation (i.e. ↑PS → ↑CO_2 elimination). **NB:** typical start-up settings are: **EPAP = 4 cm H_2O, IPAP = 12 cm H_2O (PS = IPAP – EPAP = 8 cm H_2O).** The IPAP (but NOT EPAP) can be uptitrated in increments of 2 cm H_2O to aid ventilation and ↓PCO_2 (after ABG assessment). A common mistake is to ↑IPAP and ↑EPAP together (PS remains unchanged). The FiO_2 can also be set. 💀 Patients on NIV with Type 2 ☠ should have target O_2 sats of 88–92% ONLY; titrate FiO_2 appropriately 💀. NIV is usually 'patient-triggered', but there is an adjustable 'back-up rate', which will deliver mandatory breathes, if the patient's RR drops. The rate at which the pressure ↑s from EPAP to IPAP (rise time) and the time taken for inspiration (inspiratory times) can also be altered.

Newer ventilators can deliver varying volumes breath-by-breath, as required by the patient. For example: (1) **Adaptive** servo-ventilation (ASV), used for Cheyne–Stokes respiration – it learns the patient's respiratory pattern to avoid over-ventilation by only ↑PS during the hypoventilation phase; (2) **Volume-assured pressure support (VAPS)** allows the PS to be automatically adjusted on a breath-by-breath basis (according to patient need) thereby maintaining a fixed tidal volume.

SETTING UP NIV FOR ACUTE TYPE 2 RESPIRATORY FAILURE

Top tips before commencing NIV:

- Any decision to start NIV should only follow a period of closely monitored standard medical therapy, inc the use of controlled O_2 therapy. Many patients will improve and not require NIV.
- Always consider whether invasive ventilation is the preferred option (NEVER delay intubation in favour of NIV).
- Consider whether the patient is in fact dying. NIV will not influence the inevitable outcome but may prolong suffering.
- Consider all contraindications to NIV (Table 4.1). Most are not absolute and should be considered in context (e.g. when intubation is unsuitable).
- Discuss Rx with patients (± relatives): document clearly ceiling of care, resuscitation decisions and whether intubation and mechanical ventilation will/will not be attempted should NIV fail.
- Ensure adequate monitoring (continuous RR, PR, O_2 sats and intermittent BP as a minimum), appropriately trained nursing staff and access to the correct medical bed (e.g. respiratory ward, HDU or ITU).
- Ensure Rx for the underlying condition is continued while on NIV (e.g. nebulisers); too often this is forgotten or withheld while on NIV!

Steps:

1. Select appropriate interface. Options include full face mask (preferred but less comfortable with risk of nasal bridge sores), nasal pillows (limits pressures settings, pressure can leak at mouth) and total face mask.

Table 4.1 Common indications and contraindications to NIV

Some common indications	Contraindications
Acute exacerbation of COPD (pH < 7.3)	Post-cardiac or respiratory arrest or apnoea
Acute cardiogenic pulmonary oedema	↓GCS (unable to maintain airway)
Decompensated OSA/Obesity hypoventilation	Confusion (relative; not cooperative)
Neuromuscular weakness	Severe life-threatening hypoxaemia
CAP	↑respiratory secretions
Exacerbations of bronchiectasis	Haemodynamically unstable (relative)
ILD (with reversible element, e.g. infection)	Facial deformity, trauma, burns or surgery
Bridge to transplantation in CF	Upper airway obstruction
	Pneumothorax (ALWAYS drain first to avoid tension PTx)
	Vomiting, bowel obstruction or recent upper GI surgery
	Asthma (relative; only in ITU setting and never delay intubation)

2. Explain to patient: 'Unusual pressure sensation but you will get used to it with time'.

3. Set up the ventilator. Acute NIV is delivered in **Pressure Support Mode**. ALWAYS consult local guidelines (where available). As a guide, typical initial settings for an acute exacerbation of COPD are:
   - **EPAP** = 4 cmH$_2$O
   - **IPAP** = 12 cmH$_2$O (4 IPAP – EPAP = PS of 8 cmH$_2$O)
   - **Back-up rate** = 15 breaths/min
   - **Inspiratory: Expiratory (I:E) ratio** = 1:3 (**NB**: this is achieved by setting the inspiratory time (**T$_i$**) to 1 second when the back-up is 15 breaths/min. COPD patients may require longer expiration (consider shorter Ti; typical range 0.8–1.2 seconds)
   - **FiO$_2$** = guided by the pre-NIV O$_2$ and to target sats of 88–92%. Where possible, use very little/no O$_2$. ☠ AVOID

over-oxygenation (i.e. sats > 92%) as this might ↑CO_2
further ☠

- A **higher EPAP** ≈ 8 cmH_2O may occasionally be required
  (e.g. for obesity) but always ensure adequate PS (i.e. also
  ↑IPAP)
- A faster **rise time** (300–600 ms) may be required to achieve
  synchrony if very tachypnoeic or severely obstructed.
  (**NB**: as breath/volume delivered more quickly this can be
  uncomfortable for some.)

4. Hold, or allow patient to hold the mask to face without
   attaching head straps (improves compliance).
5. Strap mask to face, but avoid excessive tightness (uncomfortable
   and likely to lead to ulceration of nasal bridge). Ideally should
   be able to fit 1–2 fingers under the straps. Check for any large
   air leaks.
6. Increase IPAP in increments of 2–5 cmH_2O over 20–30 min, until
   ≈ 20 mmH_2O (as tolerated by patient) to achieve an adequate
   tidal volume clinically (Vt also reported by many NIV machines).
7. Ensure patient adequately monitored (comfort, continuous RR,
   PR, O_2 sats and intermittent BP as a minimum).
8. Reassess immediately if there is any clinical deterioration,
   otherwise after 1 h (troubleshoot as discussed hereunder):
   - Vital signs (including GCS)
   - Chest expansion on NIV
   - Any signs of leaks
   - Repeat ABG
9. Optimal duration for NIV in acute type 2 ☠ is unknown.
   Usually use NIV until no longer acidotic and for minimum of
   24 h before weaning or discontinuing. NIV does NOT need to be
   continuous (allow breaks for drinks/meals, if clinical condition
   allows). Weaning is preferred over abrupt discontinuation
   (esp following prolonged periods of use or chronic respiratory
   failure). This is achieved by allowing supervised and extending
   periods without NIV (2–4 h at a time) during the daytime over
   approximately 48 h. Nocturnal NIV is maintained initially,

Table 4.2 NIV troubleshooting

Problem	Checks and solutions
PCO_2 ($\pm$ acidosis) remains high	Mask fits and no circuit leaks?
	Patient-NIV synchrony?
	Expiration valve patent?
	FiO_2 not inappropriately high (i.e. sats > 92%)?
	Expiratory time too short?
	Otherwise ↑PS by ↑IPAP
PO_2 remains low (< 7 kPa)	↑FiO_2 by small increments until O_2 sats 88–92%
	Consider ↑EPAP (ensure PS maintained – ↑IPAP by same amount)
Sudden clinical deterioration	No circuit leaks?
	Complication? (e.g. pneumothorax, sputum plugging or aspiration)
Hypotension	Reduce IPAP $\pm$ EPAP if tolerated
Nasal bridge irritation	Try cushion dressing or change mask type
Irritated eyes	Ensure mask fit and no leaks
Vomiting	Should NIV be discontinued?
	Consider gastric decompression with NG tube
Nasal congestion	Decongestant

but its withdrawal is the last step. Some patients do not wean successfully and require discussion with a specialist ventilation centre and consideration of domiciliary NIV.

DOMICILIARY NIV FOR CHRONIC TYPE 2 RESPIRATORY FAILURE

Domiciliary NIV has a well-established role in chronic type 2 respiratory failure due to neuromuscular weakness (e.g. scoliosis, MND, post-polio and muscular dystrophy). Nocturnal hypoventilation is most common (overnight O_2 sats < 88% or early morning PCO_2 > 6 kPa) and usually precedes daytime ✖. NIV is therefore only usually given overnight initially. Nocturnal NIV also improves daytime ventilation by 'resetting' central respiratory drive and resting respiratory muscles. The decision to commence NIV is complex and must take appropriateness (e.g. progressive nature of condition) and symptoms (morning headaches, hypersomnolence and fatigue) into consideration. Domiciliary NIV increasingly used for other causes of chronic type 2 respiratory failure, including: central hypoventilation, Cheyne–Stokes respiration, obesity hypoventilation, chronic stable COPD (with evidence of respiratory failure) and CF (as a 'bridge' to transplantation).

CONTINUOUS POSITIVE AIRWAY PRESSURE (CPAP) FOR ACUTE TYPE 1 RESPIRATORY FAILURE

Supplies a constant positive pressure across both phases of respiration (inspiration and expiration). It is effectively equivalent to the positive end expiratory pressure (PEEP) delivered by invasive ventilation. It 'splints' open (i.e. recruits) collapsed airways in order to improve VQ mismatch. Settings are usually between 5 and 10 mmH_2O with an FiO_2 that ensures adequate oxygenation, i.e. O_2 sats > 92% (PO_2 > 8 kPa). Often used for many causes of acute type 1 respiratory failure (e.g. LVF, severe pneumonia). CPAP is also used as the mainstay of Rx for OSA (page 222). Acute type 1 respiratory that is not adequately treated with high-flow oxygen alone can also be managed with newer high-flow nasal cannula devices (Optiflow™ Airvo™) (page 177).

PLEURAL EFFUSION AND THORACIC ULTRASOUND

A common manifestation of a wide range of respiratory *and* non-respiratory conditions. Most patients do NOT require a chest drain and can be managed as outpatients or on a day-case unit, where diagnostic (± therapeutic) procedures may be possible. Only the very unwell patients (e.g. hypoxic) or those with specific indications requiring a chest drain need admission. **NB:** a good quality PA CXR only detects effusions > 200 mL; USS (or lateral CXR) are more sensitive!

CAUSES OF PLEURAL EFFUSION

Commonest causes in the UK: cardiac failure, pneumonia (parapneumonic or empyema), malignancy and PE. When confronted with a pleural effusion, the FIRST and MOST IMPORTANT distinction to make is whether it is a transudate or exudate! See Box 4.4.1 and Table 4.3.

4.4.1 Transudate or exudate?

In patients with a *normal serum protein*:

- **Transudate** = pleural fluid protein < 30 g/L
- **Exudate** = pleural fluid protein > 30 g/L

In patients with a *serum protein level outside of the normal range or with borderline pleural fluid protein levels (i.e. 25–35 g/L)*, then apply **Light's criteria:** an effusion is an exudate if it meets ONE of the following criteria:

- Pleural fluid protein/serum protein ratio > 0.5
- Pleural fluid LDH/serum LDH ratio > 0.6
- Pleural fluid LDH > 2/3rd the upper limit of normal serum LDH

NB: Light's criteria are very sensitive, except in patient with cardiac failure on diuretics. A distinction between an exudate or transudate can also be made clinically (Hx & examination).

DIAGNOSTIC ALGORITHM FOR PLEURAL EFFUSION

Follow algorithm (Figure 4.3). A good history, clinical examination and CXR can identify the likely aetiology of most pleural effusions. **NB:** if there is an obvious cause for a transudate (e.g. cardiac failure) and clinical examination and CXR ± USS support this (e.g. peripheral oedema, bilateral effusions and no nodules on US), then further diagnostic procedures are NOT immediately required; start Rx and reassess response. All other cases require a **diagnostic aspiration!** (Box 4.4.2) Most exudates require a **contrast-enhanced CT thorax. Pleural biopsy** is reserved for when the cause is not apparent after CT, or histological confirmation required.

Table 4.3 Causes of pleural effusion

Transudates		Exudates	
Common causes		**Common causes**	
LVF	Only lx if atypical features	Parapneumonic	Commonest exudate in young patients
Liver cirrhosis	Often right-sided	Malignancy	Commonest exudate in older (> 60) patients
Hypoalbuminaemia	E.g. nephrotic syndrome	TB	Lymphocytic effusions (smear +ve < 5%, culture +ve only 20%, histology ≈ 100%)
Peritoneal dialysis	↑glucose content	Empyema	pH < 7.2 and features of infection
Atelectasis	Usually small		
Less common causes		**Less common causes**	
PE	Only ≈15% are transudates	PE	>80% are exudates
Hypothyroidism	Usually gross oedema	Rare infection	Viral, fungal or parasitic
Constrictive pericarditis		RA	↓glucose (< 1.6 mmol/L)
Malignancy	Rarely (< 5%) are transudates	SLE	
Meig's syndrome	With ovarian or other pelvic tumours (usually Rt-sided)	Other autoimmune conditions	E.g. Churg–Strauss, Wegener's, Sjögren's, scleroderma, dermatomyositis
Mitral stenosis		Sarcoidosis	Rare

(Continued)

Table 4.3 Causes of pleural effusion (*Continued*)

Transudates		Exudates	
Common causes		*Common causes*	
Urinothorax	Retroperitoneal leak from obstructive urinary tract (pleural fluid ↑creatinine)	**Abdominal abscess (hepatic, splenic or subphrenic)**	
		Oesophageal rupture	Can convert to empyema
		Pancreatitis	↑Amylase in pleural fluid
		Post-surgery	E.g. CABG
		Radiotherapy	Small effusions
		Uraemia	Resolve with dialysis
		Chylothorax	Chylomicrons or ↑TG
		Yellow nail syndrome	Rare triad: effusion, yellow dystrophic nails, lymphoedema (± bronchiectasis)
		Asbestosis	Benign or associated with mesothelioma
		Drugs	E.g. amiodarone, β-blockers, bromocriptine
		Rare	COP, amyloidosis and familial Mediterranean fever

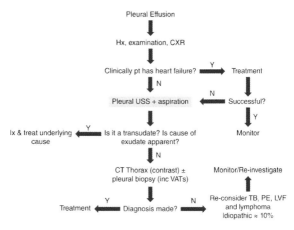

Figure 4.3 Diagnostic algorithm for pleural effusion.

4.4.2 Top Tips – Pleural fluid analysis

- Visual inspection of pleural fluid can give vital clues (e.g. pus or blood stained)
- The single most important test is pleural fluid protein
- Always tailor tests to suspected cause (some test/results can be misleading)
- Diuretics may influence the protein content of a transudate (↑)
- ↓pH usually suggest empyema but can be associated extensive malignancy or RA
- Culture of parapneumonic effusions will often be sterile
- Always suspect TB (or malignancy), if microscopy is heavily lymphocytic (e.g. > 80%)
- The yield of AFB stain and TB culture is low from pleural fluid – consider additional test, e.g. adenosine deaminase and/or pleural biopsy
- Send large volumes for cytology if malignancy is suspected

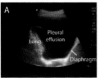 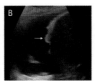 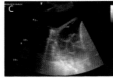

Thoracic ultrasound appearances of:

A. Pleural effusion   B. Pleural effusion with nodule   C. Loculated pleural effusion

Figure 4.4 Examples of thoracic ultrasound.

Thoracic ultrasound (TUS)

TUS is useful for the assessment of the pleural space and thorax (Box 4.4.3). It is highly recommended for ALL pleural procedures[BTS]. It can help diagnostically and may influence the management plan (e.g. diaphragmatic nodularity suggestive of malignancy). Always follow the Royal College of Radiology. Level 1 syllabus for TUS. For examples of thoracic ultrasound see Figure 4.4.

4.4.3 Importance of thoracic ultrasound

- Increases safety of pleural procedures
- Confirms effusion and rules out other causes of CXR appearance
- Can reveal complexity of an effusion (e.g. pleural thickening and/or loculation)
- Identifies additional pathology (e.g. large tumour, underlying consolidation or pleural nodules suggesting metastases)

PLEURODESIS

Chemical pleurodesis is used to prevent the recurrence of pleural effusions (typically malignant) or PTx (less commonly; only if NOT suitable for surgery). Sclerosants seal the visceral pleura against the parietal pleura by inducing adhesions → prevents re-accumulation of air (PTx) or fluid (effusion). They are usually instilled via an intercostal drain or during surgery. **Talc (4 g STERITALC®)** is the most effective. A slurry is prepared in normal saline prior to use.

4.5.1 Top Tips

- Successful pleurodesis more likely if drainage is complete, i.e. lung fully re-expanded with apposition of pleural surfaces:
  - Once drain output < 150 mL/24 h, confirm complete drainage on CXR (± US if uncertainty)
  - Pleural apposition can be further encouraged with suction (discussed hereunder)
- Anti-inflammatory drugs may prevent the pleural inflammatory response and generation of adhesions → if possible stop corticosteroids (or NSAIDs) or delay pleurodesis until course complete.
- Pleurodesis is painful! → use intrapleural local anaesthesia (discussed hereunder), opiate premedication (± sedation) and regular analgesia after the procedure.

PROCEDURE

Most hospitals have a protocol (please consult). Talc is unlicensed and needs to be prescribed and ordered from pharmacy on a named patient basis. Recommended protocol:

1. Ensure complete drainage and lung re-expansion (discussed earlier)
2. Administer appropriate analgesia (e.g. oramorph)
3. Ensure patent chest drain (i.e. swinging with respiration ± gentle flush if uncertain)
4. Prepare sterile Talc slurry:
   - Shake Talc vial (4 g) to break up powder
   - Draw up 30 mL of normal saline and inject into Talc vial
   - Gently reconstitute powder (avoid shaking), then draw up into 50 mL leur lock syringe

5. Administer intrapleural 1% lignocaine (10 mg/mL): instil 3 mg/kg into chest drain (e.g. 21 mL for 70 kg; max. 250 mg [25 mL])
6. Clamp drain (or close 3-way tap) for a few minimum
7. Administer Talc slurry via chest drain, followed immediately by 20 mL of normal saline flush
8. Clamp drain (or close 3-way tap) for 1 h and encourage patient to roll into different positions
9. Open drain to allow drainage; some advocate the use of suction (approx. 20 mm H_2O)
10. Closely monitor patient during and after pleurodesis (complications as discussed hereunder)
11. Aim to remove drain after 24 h

🕮 **Complications:** Pain, fever and rarely ARDS (< 1%) 🕮.

PULMONARY MANIFESTATIONS OF CONNECTIVE TISSUE DISEASE

Patients with connective tissue disease are often referred with pulmonary manifestations or associations. It is important to consider the adverse effects of any immunosuppressant (e.g. methotrexate (Box 4.6.1) or anti-TNF-α (Box 4.6.2); discussed hereunder) and infection (2° to immunosuppression – may be atypical, e.g. PCP, TB, NTM, fungal, CMV). Consider the following investigations: autoantibodies, CXR ± HRCT, sputum MC&S (inc. AAFB), lung function tests, bronchoscopy + BAL (MC&S, AAFB, PCP) + transbronchial biopsy and surgical lung biopsy (rarely).

4.6.1 Methotrexate and pneumonitis

Occurs in 5% of those Rx with methotrexate. Usually subacute (≤ 4 months of starting) with cough, SOB, ↑T° and widespread crackles. Can be more acute. Life-threatening (20% mortality). Lung function is restrictive, CXR/CT → infiltration, ↑blood EΦ, ↑BAL LΦ. **Rx:** stop methotrexate + corticosteroids (prednisolone or iv methylprednisolone).

4.6.2 Anti-TNF-α therapy and MTB

Anti-TNF-α therapy (e.g. infliximab, etanercept, adalimumab, rituximab) predisposes to infection, inc viral, fungal and opportunistic (PCP, TB and NTM). ↑risk of malignancy and may worsen ILD. ALWAYS screen for MTB before starting Rx (i.e. Hx, examination, CXR and TST/IGRA). Current guidance[BTS/NICE]:

1 Rx active MTB for ≥ 2 months before starting anti-TNF-α.
2 For those with a previous Hx of MTB:
   If received *adequate* MTB Rx → start anti-TNF-α and monitor every 3 months.
   If received *inadequate* MTB Rx → exclude active MTB before starting MTB chemoprophylaxis.
3 Risk assess all others:
   ↓*risk* (e.g. white British, normal CXR, negative TST) safe to start anti-TNF-α.
   ↑*risk* (e.g. black African, South Asian, positive TST) give MTB chemoprophylaxis concurrently.
4 Advise all patients on Sx of MTB: if patient develops MTB → Rx with standard regimen and can continue anti-TNF-α.

RHEUMATOID ARTHRITIS

Chronic deforming symmetrical peripheral arthropathy with non-articular manifestations. Important pulmonary associations include:

- **Nodules:** Seropositive disease only. Usually incidental and asymptomatic (rarely cause pneumothorax or haemoptysis). Single or multiple, mainly subpleural or along interlobular septa. Differentiate from lung cancer; stable size on CT, mild/no uptake on PET-CT, benign biopsy.
- **Fibrosis:** Tends to occur in seropositive ± multi-system disease ± male smokers. Similar to IPF/UIP: Clubbing, restrictive lung function, subpleural/basal reticular pattern. Try steroids ± immunosuppressants (often ineffective). Pneumonitis (± methotrexate) is less common.
- **Bronchiectasis:** Common (1/3rd RA).

- **Pleural disease:** Effusions are common but usually small and asymptomatic; may require drainage ± steroids. Pleuritic pain from pleuritic is common.
- **Organising pneumonia:** See page 92. Responds to steroids.
- **Caplan's syndrome:** Rare; combination of RA, nodules and coal-worker's pneumoconiosis.
- **Small airways disease:** Airway obstruction and hyperinflation (1/3rd RA), less commonly obliterative bronchiolitis. May be rapidly progressive and irreversible. Rx with steroids (po, ± high-dose ICS). May need to consider transplant.
- **Cricoarytenoid arthritis:** Can cause sore throat, hoarse voice, stridor, OSA. Usually Rx with steroids (po, or joint injection).

SYSTEMIC LUPUS ERYTHEMATOSUS

Multi-system autoimmune disease with ↑dsDNA titres. Pulmonary disease is very common and may be presenting feature:

- **Pleural disease:** Effusion and pleuritis (pain ± rub) are common. Need to exclude other causes. Rx = NSAIDs and steroids.
- **Fibrosis:** Most commonly resembles RA-associated fibrosis (discussed earlier). Usually mild/asymptomatic. Rarely acute lupus pneumonitis (severe and life-threatening).
- **PE:** Most common with ↑antiphospholipid antibodies.
- **PHT:** Very poor prognosis.
- **Alveolar haemorrhage:** Rare but life-threatening. Rx = steroids + cyclophosphamide.
- **Shrinking lung syndrome:** Very rare. Restrictive lung disease with normal lung parenchyma caused by diaphragmatic weakness.

SYSTEMIC SCLEROSIS

Systemic autoimmune disease characterised by ↑ deposition of connective tissue macromolecules in skin and other organs + fibroproliferative changes in the microvasculature. Skin is classically thick, tight and shiny skin (hands, face and neck). Can present as *limited cutaneous disease* (**CREST** syndrome: **C**alcinosis, **R**aynauds, o**E**sophageal **D**ysmotility, **S**clerodactyly, and <u>T</u>elangiectasia), *diffuse cutaneous disease, sine scleroderma* (absent skin changes) or as an *overlap syndrome* (with SLE, RA or polymyositis). Lung complications are the usual cause of death:

- **Fibrosis:** Very common. Either NSIP or IPF (UIP) pattern. Many are SOB with restrictive lung function + ↓kCO. Rx with cyclophosphamide and steroids.
- **PHT:** May be secondary to fibrosis or isolated. Rx is with prostacyclin infusion. Transplantation may be required.
- **Bronchiectasis:** Often mild.
- **Aspiration:** From oesophageal dysmotility. May cause pneumonia ± play a role in fibrosis and bronchiectasis.
- **Chronic organising pneumonia:** See page 92.
- **Hide-bound chest:** Restricted chest expansion from tight skin on chest (very rare).

POLY/DERMATOMYOSITIS

Symmetrical proximal muscle weakness with ↑CK and EMG changes. Dermatomyositis has additional skin features (Gottron's papules, Heliotrope and erythematous rashes). Important lung complications include:

- **Ventilatory failure:** Secondary to weakness of diaphragm ± intercostal muscle.
- **Interstitial lung disease:** Many different processes are reported: UIP, NSIP, COP, vasculitis with haemorrhage. Fibrosis may be associated with PHT or rarely spontaneous pneumomediastinum. Fibrosis may require steroid and cyclophosphamide Rx. *Antisynthetase syndrome* is rare and characterized by poly/ dermatomyositis, ↑antisynthetase antibodies, ↑T°, arthritis, Raynaud's phenomenon, mechanic's hands and ILD.
- **Aspiration pneumonia:** Arises from pharyngeal muscle weakness.

SJÖGREN'S SYNDROME

Systemic chronic inflammatory disorder characterised by lymphocytic infiltration of exocrine organs → sicca symptoms, e.g. xerophthalmia (dry eyes), xerostomia (dry mouth), and parotid gland enlargement. Secondary Sjögren's is associated with connective tissue disease (e.g. RA). Lung involvement occurs in ≈ 25%:

- **Pleural:** Pleuritic chest pain, thickening and effusion.
- **Xerotrachea:** Atrophy of mucus glands causing a chronic dry cough and recurrent infection.
- **Airways disease:** Usually only mild obstructive disease (hyper-reactivity, bronchitis).
- **Diffuse interstitial disease:** Usually mild/asymptomatic. May resemble NSIP, LIP, UIP. Pneumonitis and organising pneumonia are also seen.
- **Lymphoma:** More common in Sjögren's.

ANKYLOSING SPONDYLITIS

Chronic inflammatory arthritis affecting axial skeleton and sacroiliac joints. Pulmonary manifestations include:

- **Restrictive lung disease:** From costovertebral deformity and rigidity.
- **Fibrosis:** Typically bilateral and apical.

PULMONARY REHABILITATION

Pulmonary rehabilitation (PR) is an evidence-based multidisciplinary approach that targets the extrapulmonary manifestations of chronic lung disease (esp ↓muscle mass). PR improves muscle function and interrupts the vicious cycle of inactivity due SOB and deconditioning. Highly cost effective Rx for COPD → ↑exercise tolerance, ↑QoL and ↓rates and length of hospitalisation. Now also used for many chronic lung conditions.

PROGRAMME

Run on an outpatient basis (often in the community) by a multidisciplinary team (frequently led by physiotherapists), typically over a 6-wk period. Comprises:

1. **Physical training:** Main component is an individualised high-intensity aerobic exercise programme, e.g. cycling 2–3 times/wk

with additional wkly classes. Upper and lower limb strength training (with weights) is often included. O_2 can be provided for patients who desaturate.

2. **Disease education**
3. **Nutritional education**
4. **Psychosocial intervention:** Including advice or Rx for anxiety, depression and smoking cessation.
5. **Refresher course:** Benefits of PR lost 6–12 months after course completion. On-going sessions may offer sustained benefits.

Outcomes from PR are formally assessed using measures of exercise tolerance (e.g. shuttle walk or 6MWT) and disease-specific questionnaires (e.g. SGRQ).

SLEEP APNOEA AND HYPOVENTILATION

There are two types of sleep apnoea: (1) **Obstructive Sleep Apnoea (OSA)**; caused by dynamic upper airway obstruction during sleep and (2) **Central Sleep Apnoea (CSA)**; ↓ventilation during sleep without upper airway obstruction (many causes; discussed hereunder). OSA is by far the most common ($\approx 85\%$ sleep-disordered breathing). Some patients can have both.

OBSTRUCTIVE SLEEP APNOEA (OSA)

Some URT narrowing is normal during sleep, as all postural muscles relax (inc. pharyngeal dilators). Excessive narrowing can occur with ↑ soft tissue (e.g. obese, muscular, hypothyroid, large tonsils), craniofacial abnormalities (even subtle), neuromuscular disease and use of muscle relaxants (esp. sedatives or alcohol). The spectrum ranges from 'unobtrusive snoring' to numerous episodes of complete airflow obstruction. Sleep may as a result be sufficiently fragmented to cause daytime symptoms, inc. somnolence and may require intervention (Box 4.8.1). OSA is an important risk factor for hypertension and cardio-/cerebrovascular disease.

4.8.1 A basic guide to OSA assessment in clinic

- Assess severity of sleepiness using the **Epworth Sleepiness Scale (ESS)**
- Obtain history of snoring ± apnoea (best from witness, e.g. spouse)
- Ask about associated symptoms (e.g. ↓concentration, nocturia, ↓libido, GORD)
- Ask about relevant PMH (e.g. ENT surgery)
- Check for endocrinological disease (e.g. hypothyroid, acromegaly, Cushing's, DM)
- Check for cardiovascular/cerebrovascular risk factors (may ↓threshold for OSA Rx)
- Alcohol history and use of sedatives (exacerbating factors)
- Occupation (may have implications for vigilance and/or driving)
- Check BMI and neck circumference (> 17 inches for men correlates with OSA)
- Examine oropharynx (**Mallampati**; discussed hereunder) and mandible (often small and set-back)
- Assess for coexisting respiratory conditions (e.g. CXR + spirometry)
- Other tests if indicated (e.g. ABG if ❀ suspected, TSH, FBC, U&E, BM, HbA1c, chol or TG)

Sleep studies

Vary between centres. Include: (1) overnight oximetry – O_2 sats with PR; (2) 'limited' or respiratory polysomnography (PSG) – overnight oximetry with addition of sound, oronasal flows, chest, abdominal and limb movements; (3) Full PSG – addition of electro-encephalogram/-oculogram/-myogram (rarely used for OSA diagnosis). (1) and (2) are the most commonly deployed. **NB:** thresholds for defining OSA pathology (e.g. apnoea or AHI) are arbitrary. Large grey areas exist between disease and normality (Figure 4.5). Results can vary significantly from night-to-night. Decisions to Rx should therefore NOT be based on sleep study results alone. Where sleep studies are equivocal, it may be appropriate to undertake a therapeutic trial of CPAP.

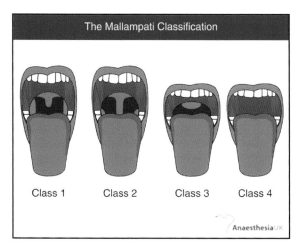

Figure 4.5 Mallampati Classification. Class 1: full visibility of tonsils, uvula and soft palate; Class 2: visibility of hard and soft palate, upper portion of tonsils and uvula; Class 3: soft and hard palate and base of uvula are visible; Class 4: only hard palate visible.

4.8.2 Epworth Sleepiness Scale Questionnaire

How likely are you to doze off or fall asleep in the following situations, in contrast to feeling just tired? This refers to your usual way of life in recent times. Even if you have not done some of these things recently, try to work out how they would have affected you. Use the following scale to choose the most appropriate number for each situation:

0 = would never doze 1 = slight chance of dozing
2 = moderate chance of dozing
3 = high chance of dozing

Sitting and reading?	0	1	2	3
Watching TV?	0	1	2	3

Sitting inactive in a public place (e.g. a theatre or meeting)?	0	1	2	3
As a passenger in a car for an hour without a break?	0	1	2	3
Lying down to rest in the afternoon when circumstances permit?	0	1	2	3
Sitting and talking to someone?	0	1	2	3
Sitting quietly after a lunch without alcohol?	0	1	2	3
In a car, while stopped for a few minutes in traffic?	0	1	2	3

Total = 24 (Score ≥ 11 suggestive of excessive daytime sleepiness)

(11–14 = mild; 15–18 = moderate; 19–24 = severe)

Reproduced from Murray W. Johns – A New Method for Measuring Daytime Sleepiness: The Epworth Sleepiness Scale – Sleep 1991; 14: 540–545.

Some important definitions from a limited PSG:

- **Apnoea** = complete cessation of airflow lasting ≥ 10 s
- **Hypopnoea** = ↓ airflow (> 50%) lasting ≥ 10 s + O_2 desaturation (discussed hereunder) or evidence of sleep fragmentation/arousal.
- **Apnoea Hypopnoea Index (AHI)** = no. of events (apnoea or hypopnoea) per hour of sleep. **AHI < 5/h** considered normal; **5–14/h** = mild OSA; **15–29/h** = moderate OSA; **≥ 30/h** = severe.
- **OSA** = AHI ≥ 5/h + symptoms of sleep-disordered breathing
- **Oxygen desaturation** = most common definition is ≥ 4% drop in O_2 sats. Multiple sawtooth-shaped (slow fall/quick rise) O_2 desaturations are indicative of OSA.
- **Oxygen desaturation index (ODI)** = no. of O_2 desaturation events/h of sleep; correlates with AHI. 'Cut-off' values vary between centres (**ODI > 10/h** usually considered significant). The time spent hypoxic (e.g. Sats < 90%) ± the degree of hypoxia are likely to be just as important.

Treatment

Discuss options with the patient. Not all patients require Rx; symptoms rather than abnormal sleep reports should drive decisions to Rx, as should effects on QoL, patient profession, wishes/motivation, evidence of ✖ and cardio-/cerebrovascular risk/disease.

Simple measures: For all patients with OSA consider referral to a dietician and advising weight loss (often not achievable or maintained in practise), ↓alcohol (esp. evening), sleeping decubitus, raising the head of the bed, Rx for GORD (e.g. 20 mg omeprazole po od) and nasal congestion (e.g. fluticasone 55 mcg each nostril od [AVAMYS®]).

Snorers ± mild OSA: Mandibular advancement devices (MADs) displace the mandible anteriorly (like a 'jaw-thrust'). Often trialled for snorers (minimal/no OSA), mild OSA without significant daytime Sx and patients who can't tolerate CPAP. NOT recommended for severe OSA, respiratory failure or excessive symptoms. They require adequate dentition. MADs fitted by a dentist are preferable: DIY devices exist. Evidence for effectiveness is limited. MADs may be useful, esp. for those with a set-back mandible. SE inc. tooth/jaw pain and ↑salivation.

Pharyngeal surgery: Discouraged – used as a last resort, e.g. mandibular/maxillary advancement surgery for significant OSA.

Sleep position training: Important for patients with supine-only OSA. Belts can be worn to help position the patient on their side during sleep.

CPAP: is mainstay of Rx for 'Significant' OSA. Delivers pressure (usually 5–10 cm H_2O) to splint open the URT, preventing collapse, sleep fragmentation, consequent daytime Sxs and ↑QoL. Support from a technician/specialist nurse helps ↑ compliance. NIV may be required where there is respiratory failure (↑CO_2), long-term or for a short period before switching to CPAP.

Pharmacotherapy: Some evidence that the addition of 'alerting drugs' (i.e. modafinil 200 mg po od) may ↑ sleepiness in some patients who remain sleepy despite adequate CPAP compliance. NOT a routine Rx and only to be prescribed by specialist!

4.8.3 Driving with OSA

Always consult the DVLA website for the latest advice:

- https://www.gov.uk/government/publications/at-a-glance
- https://www.gov.uk/obstructive-sleep-apnoea-and-driving

It is the doctor's duty to explain to the patient that we are responsible for our own levels of vigilance while driving and that no one should drive while they are sleepy, regardless of the underlying cause; a prison sentence can result from a sleep-related accident!

A patient should stop driving and write to the DVLA if they experience daytime symptoms that could impair driving ability. They will be asked to complete the SL1 or SL1V questionnaire.

Patients should not drive if they experience excessive daytime sleepiness (regardless of whether they are treated).

A patient can continue/resume driving if:

They are not sleepy (even if they meet OSA criteria on a sleep study)

Sleepiness has resolved with Rx, e.g. CPAP (advised to gain medical confirmation)

They are class 2 licence-holders, but successful Rx has been verified by a specialist clinic (often > 3 h CPAP/night and normal ESS)

The DVLA requires drivers with OSA to be reviewed every 3 years (Group 1) or annually (Group 2).

CENTRAL SLEEP APNOEA (CSA)

Much less common than OSA. Ranges from inability to adequately expand the chest for inspiration through to loss of central ventilatory drive. The underlying cause(s) is often apparent from detailed clinical assessment (e.g. Hx, examination and lung function). Most commonly results from one, or a combination of:

1. ↓**Ventilatory drive** $2°$ to brainstem damage (e.g. stroke, tumour, syringobulbia, congenital).

2. **Respiratory pump failure** $2°$ to weak inspiratory muscles. Respiration becomes more dependent on the accessory muscles as a neuromuscular conditions progresses. During sleep, however, these muscles are hypotonic/atonic. The metabolic ventilatory drive is able to deliver 'rescue ventilation' but at the cost of recurrent arousals and ↓sleep quality.

3. **Palsy of the diaphragm,** the only functioning respiratory muscle during REM sleep.

4. **Restrictive chest wall disease,** e.g. scoliosis (inspiratory muscles mechanically disadvantaged).

5. **Obesity Hypoventilation Syndrome (OHS)** is defined as an awake hypercapnia ($PCO_2 > 6$ kPa) in a patient with a BMI > 30 kg/m^2. Results from the excessive load on the respiratory muscles and impaired ventilatory control centrally. Frequently overlaps with OSA.

6. **COPD.** Respiratory muscles are 'overloaded' due to hyperinflation → ventilation more dependent on accessory muscles, which become hypotonic/atonic during sleep.

7. **Cheyne–Stokes respiration** with LVF or altitude.

Investigation

Sleep studies can be difficult to interpret in CSA and ALWAYS require an experienced opinion, e.g. identifying the difference between 'true' apnoea *or* weak inspiratory muscles. CSA is often confirmed by regular O_2 desaturation events without any evidence of apnoeas/hypopnoea (or snoring). However, CSA does frequently overlap with OSA (e.g. in OHS). **ABG** will reveal diurnal type 2 respiratory failure (↑early-morning CO_2), metabolic alkalosis (↑HCO_3 and normal PCO_2) or progression to a compensated (↑CO_2 and ↑HCO_3) or decompensated type 2 respiratory failure (↑CO_2 and acidosis).

Treatment

Nasal O_2 can be sufficient for some patients (e.g. LVF or COPD without hypercapnia). However, nocturnal NIV is usually recommended (good practice to FIRST Rx and improve LVF for Cheyne–Stokes respiration). OHS is associated with high rates of mortality and NIV should be commenced promptly, often during the hospital admission and continued at discharge. ALWAYS seek advice from the respiratory team!

SMOKING CESSATION AND NICOTINE REPLACEMENT

Smoking is the 1° cause of COPD and lung cancer, and is an important risk factor for cardiovascular and cerebrovascular disease. Approximately 20% of the UK population smoke. Nicotine is a major component of tobacco. It activates the mesolimbic pathway and is highly addictive. Combining nicotine replacement therapy (NRT) with counselling achieves the highest quit rates. Rx should be chosen to accommodate the smoker's likely adherence, preferences, availability of counselling and support, previous experience of smoking-cessation aids, contraindications and adverse effects of the preparations[BNF] (Box 4.9.1).

Pharmacological options include NRT, bupropion or varenicline. **NB:** combining NRT with bupropion or varenicline is NOT recommended. Smokers should also have access to cessation services for behavioural support. Non-pharmacological measures should also be recommended, including **hypnotherapy** or **acupuncture**.

4.9.1 Cessation and concomitant Rx

Cigarette smoking ↑metabolism of some drugs by stimulating CYP1A2. The dose of some drugs may need to be ↓ with smoking cessation, inc theophylline, cinacalcet, ropinirole and some antipsychotics (e.g. clozapine, olanzapine, chlorpromazine, and haloperidol). Regularly monitor for adverse effects.

NICOTINE REPLACEMENT THERAPY

Mainstay of smoking cessation Rx. NRT replaces smoking after an abrupt withdrawal, helps ↓ no. of cigarettes prior to an attempt to quit and can ↓ cravings. Many preparations are available: prolonged-release transdermal patches (16 h or 24 h) or intermediate-release chewing gums, inhalation cartridges, lozenges, sublingual tablets, oral sprays and nasal sprays. Many are available over the counter. Choice depends on patient preference and should take into account any previously used preparations. Patients with a ↑ level of nicotine dependence, or who have failed with NRT previously, may benefit from combining a patch with an immediate-release preparation for urges or cravings. Please see page 32 for important cautions and side effects.

Transdermal patches: Different strengths available, released over 16 h or 24 h. Advice patient to apply on waking to dry, non-hairy skin (hip, trunk or upper arm) and hold in position for 10–20 sec for adhesion, rotating sites with each application. **Available:** *16-h preparations* – NICORETTE (5, 10, 15 mg/16 h), NICORETTE INVISI PATCH (10, 15, 25 mg/16 h) or NICASSIST (10, 15, 25 mg/16 h); *24-h preparations* – NICOTINELL (7, 14, 21 mg/24 h), NIQUITIN (7, 14, 21 mg/24 h) or NICASSIST (7, 14, 21 mg/24 h). A simple guide for use[BNF]: **> 10 cigarettes/d:** use high-strength patch for 6–8 wks → medium strength 2 wks → low strength 2 wks; **< 10 cigarettes/d:** use medium strength 6–8 wks → low strength 2–4 wks. Patch strength can be ↑ if withdrawal symptoms are experienced or abstinence not achieved/maintained.

Chewing gums: Available as 2 mg or 4 mg gums. Use with urge to smoke or to prevent cravings. The act of chewing can also ↓ cravings. Advise to chew until the taste becomes strong, then rest gum inside cheek to allow nicotine to be absorbed buccally. When the taste fades, repeat process. One piece of gum lasts for ≈ 30 min. **Available:** NICORETTE, NICASSIST, NICOTINELL or NIQUITIN (all 2 mg or 4 mg). A simple guide for use[BNF]: **< 20 cigarettes/d** → 2 mg gum (max. 15 pieces/24 h; if exceed use 4 mg gum); **> 20 cigarettes/d** → 4 mg gum. ☠ Should NOT exceed a total of 15 pieces of 4 mg/24 h ☠. Use for 3-month period before reducing strength or discontinuing.

Inhalation cartridges: Use with urge to smoke/to prevent cravings. Useful for those who are habitual smokers and find it hard to stop the 'hand-to-mouth' routine. Absorption is buccal/sublingual and not via the lungs. Available as 10 mg (20 min use) or 15 mg (40 min use) cartridges; NICORETTE or NICASSIST.

Lozenges: Use 1 lozenge every 1–2 h with the urge to smoke. Advise to allow the lozenge to dissolve slowly in the mouth while periodically moving it from one side to the other. **Available:** NICORETTE (2 mg), NICOTINELL (1, 2 mg) or NIQUITIN (1.5, 2, 4 mg). A simple guide for use[BNF]: **< 20 cigarettes/d** → lower strength; **> 20 cigarettes/d** (or failure to stop smoking) → higher strength. Maximum dose = 15 lozenges/d. Continue with lozenges for 6–12 wks before attempting ↓dose.

Sublingual tablets: Useful for smokers who want a discreet form of treatment. Advise to place tablet under tongue and allow to dissolve. **Available:** NICORETTE MICROTAB or NICASSIST MICROTAB (both 2 mg). A simple guide for use[BNF]: **< 20 cigarettes/d** → 1 tablet each hour; **> 20 cigarettes/d** (or failure to stop smoking) → 2 tablets each hour. Maximum dose 40 tablets/24 h. Continue for 3 months before attempting to ↓ dose.

Oral sprays: Advise to use 1–2 sprays with urge to smoke or to prevent cravings (do NOT exceed 4 sprays/h and 64 sprays/d). Avoid inhalation while spraying or swallowing immediately after use. Available: NICORETTE QUICKMIST (1 mg/metered dose).

Nasal sprays: Faster absorption and ↑ relief of cravings. Spray once into each nostril with the urge to smoke, up to twice/h for 16 h daily (max. 64 sprays/d). Continue for 8 wks before ↓ dose. Available: NICORETTE or NICASSIST (500 mcg/metered spray).

DRUGS USED IN NICOTINE DEPENDENCE

Bupropion (ZYBAN; page 13) and Varenicline (CHAMPIX; page 46) are drugs, which can be prescribed in nicotine dependence.

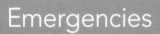

Emergencies

DOI: 10.1201/9781315151816-5

ACUTE ASTHMA

Acute asthma is diagnosed clinically (Box 5.1.1). Important alternative diagnoses include anaphylaxis or upper respiratory tract obstruction (distinguish wheeze from stridor).

Initial assessment: Try to identify 'brittle asthma' (sporadic sudden falls in PEFR in a patient who is usually well-controlled) or those presenting with, or at risk of severe/life-threatening asthma (Box 5.1.2). Other patients can often be discharged from A&E after appropriate Rx, ensuring: adequate period of observation (e.g. > 1 h after nebuliser), PEFR > 75% predicted (or 75% of best PEFR), that there are no concerns (e.g. lives alone), that Rx compliance is assessed (e.g. inhaler technique) and appropriate follow-up is arranged.

5.1.1 Important risk factors for fatal asthma

- Previous near fatal attack (e.g. ventilated) – greatest predictor
- Repeated A&E attendances or hospital admissions
- ≥ 3 classes of asthma medication
- Large amounts of β_2 agonist use
- Brittle asthma

Psychosocial features, e.g. low-socioeconomic status, illicit drug misuse, psychiatric disease

---

5.1.2 Features of severe and life-threatening asthma

Severe: If any one of:

- PEFR 33–50% predicted or best
- RR ≥ 25/min
- PR ≥ 110/min
- Inability to complete sentences in one breath

Life-threatening: If any one of:

- Poor respiratory effort
- Silent chest (signifies significant bronchoconstriction; > wheeze)

- Confusion
- Coma
- Cardiovascular compromise (arrhythmia, hypotension)
- PEFR < 33% predicted or best
- SaO_2 < 92% (also indication for ABG sampling)
- PaO_2 < 8 kPa
- $\leftrightarrow PCO_2$ (indicative of tiring patient)
- $\uparrow PCO_2$ (near fatal; urgent intubation required!)

EMERGENCY MANAGEMENT

Start Rx prior to any investigations, while patient is being assessed[BTS/SIGN]:

1. Sit patient upright
2. Administer 40–60% O_2 through high-flow mask, e.g. Hudson mask
3. Attach O_2 Sats monitor (+ cardiac leads and BP cuff)
4. Attempt to record PEFR (not always possible if significant respiratory distress)
5. Salbutamol 2.5–5 mg via O_2-driven neb given 'back to back' (repeat every 15 min if life-threatening)
6. Ipratropium 0.5 mg via O_2-driven neb (can repeat up to every 4–6 h if life-threatening or fails to respond to salbutamol)
7. Administer corticosteroids: Prednisolone 40–50 mg po od for at least 5 days *or* hydrocortisone 100 mg qds iv if unable to swallow or retain tablets. **NB:** prednisolone po considered as effective, Do *not* delay administration if cannulation difficult
8. Consider investigations: ABG if O_2 sats < 92%, blood tests and CXR (important to exclude pneumothorax)

If life-threatening features or patient failing to improve (☠ **NB:** patient may not appear distressed ☠), get senior ± ITU support early and consider the following:

1. **$MgSO_4$ ivi:** 1.2–2 g over 20 min (8 mmol = 2 g = 4 mL of 50% solution) unlicensed indication.

2. **Salbutamol ivi:** 5 microgram/kg over 10 min initially (then up to 20 microgram/min ivi according to response): 'back-to-back' nebs now often preferred (ivi rarely given).

3. **Aminophylline iv:** Attach cardiac monitor and give loading dose 5 mg/kg iv over 20 min, then ivi at 0.5–0.7 mg/kg/h (0.3 mg/kg/h if elderly). 💀 Omit loading and check levels ASAP to guide dosing if on maintenance po aminophylline/theophylline. 💀 Risk of serious arrhythmias, hypotension, vomiting and seizures. Only use on specialist advice; many will not respond and many will have SEs (difficult to predict).

4. **Adrenaline im:** Occasionally useful if peri-arrest (500 micrograms as 0.5 mL of 1:1000).

5. **Heliox:** Helium and O_2 gas mixture; requires less effort for respiration. Predominantly used for upper airway obstruction. May benefit medium airway narrowing. Specialist advice only.

💀 Never start NIV for asthmatics with hypercapnic respiratory failure on medical wards; this is a feature of life-threatening asthma and is an indication for mechanical ventilation. 💀

ACUTE RESPIRATORY DISTRESS SYNDROME (ARDS)

Acute, severe and life-threatening lung injury resulting in multiple respiratory and non-respiratory conditions (discussed hereunder) (Box 5.2.1). **Characterised by:** (1) alveolar and parenchymal inflammation (2° to locally or remotely produced mediators); (2) ↑ vascular permeability; (3) diffuse bilateral pulmonary infiltrates; (4) severe VQ mismatch with significant hypoxia (PO_2:FiO_2 ratio < 27 kPa); (5) ↓ lung compliance ('stiff lungs'); (6) absence of LVF (no clinical features *or* PAWP < 18 mmHg). Acute lung injury (ALI) is considered a 'milder' form (PaO_2:FiO_2 < 40 kPa) with similar causes.

TREATMENT

Rx underlying cause. Start high-flow O_2 via Hudson mask. Seek ITU support early → CPAP or mechanical ventilation required.

Avoid excessive use of ivi fluids ± try a diuretic (☠ sepsis/shock ☠). Ventilation strategies are designed to prevent further damage from barotrauma (↑ ventilation pressure) *or* hyperoxia, inc prone, airway pressure release ventilation (APRV), high frequency ventilation (uses ↓TV but ↑RR) and permissive hypercapnia. Some may require extracorporeal membrane oxygenation (ECMO). Pulmonary infection is a common complication →↓ threshold for antibiotics.

5.2.1 Some important causes of ARDS/ALI

- Sepsis (any, inc pulmonary)
- Aspiration
- Trauma
- Pancreatitis
- Burns (inc smoke inhalation)
- Significant blood transfusion, i.e. > 6 units (TRALI – transfusion related acute lung injury)
- Transplantation (inc pulmonary)
- Drug overdose (e.g. TCA or aspirin)
- Near drowning

ALTITUDE SICKNESS

Also known as **acute mountain sickness, altitude illness, hypobaropathy** or **'the altitude bends'**. Caused by ↓PaO_2 at high altitude (> 8000 feet or 2400 m) → ↓PO_2, hyperventilation with ↓CO_2/respiratory ↑pH and cerebral vasoconstriction. Most symptoms are nonspecific (Box 5.3.1). Can progress to **high altitude pulmonary oedema (HAPE)** ± **high altitude cerebral oedema (HACE)**; often fatal.

MANAGEMENT
Prevention[NHS]:

1. Ascend slowly (≤ 300 m or 1000 feet/24 h) with a rest every third day

5.3.1 Symptoms and signs of altitude sickness

MINOR

- Light-headed/headache
- Fatigue
- Nausea/vomiting/anorexia
- Numbness/tingling in hands and feet
- Insomnia/period nocturnal ventilation
- Peripheral oedema

MAJOR

HAPE (non-uniform pulmonary vasoconstriction $\rightarrow \uparrow$PAP):
- Cough/SOB
- Cyanosis
- Pink frothy sputum (pulmonary oedema with haemorrhage)
- Widespread crackles

HACE:
- Ataxia (early warning sign)
- Retinal haemorrhages/papilloedema/cerebral thrombosis/petechial haemorrhages
- Headache
- Confusion/disorientation/hallucinations/$\downarrow$GCS

2. Acclimatisation, e.g. 'climb high, sleep low' strategy, rise $\approx$ 300 m/day but return to a lower altitude to sleep
3. Hydration (avoid alcohol)
4. Avoid cigarette smoking
5. **Acetazolamide** (DIAMOX SR): 250 mg po bd taken for 48–72 h before ascent[CDC]. Induces a mild metabolic $\downarrow$pH to prepare for $\uparrow$RR and respiratory $\uparrow$pH

Treatment:

1. Consider urgent descent
2. $\uparrow$FiO$_2$ with supplement O$_2$ and/or a Gamow bag (portable and inflatable pressure bag that accommodates one person)

3. Start acetazolamide (DIAMOX SR)
4. Nifedipine 20 mg po qds to ↓PAP in HAPE
5. Dexamethasone 4 mg po qds (load with 8 mg) with HACE

ANAPHYLAXIS

Anaphylaxis: Allergic/immunological, IgE-mediated, type 1 hypersensitivity, multi-system reaction rapidly resulting from allergen exposure, which can inc drug ingestion (esp parenteral penicillin), a bee or wasp sting, latex or foods such as nuts and seafood.

Non-IgE-mediated, non-allergic anaphylaxis: Clinically identical reaction, most commonly following radio-contrast media, or aspirin/NSAID exposure. Not triggered by IgE antibodies. Previously termed 'anaphylactoid reaction'.

Treatment: Both are treated in the *same* way. **See anaphylaxis algorithm inside front cover.**

First-line Rx includes high flow O_2, adrenaline im (0.5 mL of 1:1000), salbutamol neb 2.5–5 mg (± neb adrenaline 1:1000 diluted to 4 mL in sodium chloride 0.9%), fluids (if signs of shock), hydrocortisone 200 mg iv and chlorphenamine 10 mg iv (over 1 min) or im. ☠ Remember to remove the allergen (e.g. stop drug infusion). ☠

Discharge and follow-up: Provide adrenaline im for self-administration (EPIPEN). Consider referral to immunology, esp if allergen not identified or repeated episodes. Allergen immunotherapy (desensitisation) may help those with specific IgE to an allergen causing repeated anaphylaxis.

Hereditary angioedema: Suspect if repeated attacks of oedema to the face, upper respiratory tract (laryngeal → intubate), periphery or GI tract (mimics bowel obstruction). Often triggered, e.g. by surgery, trauma, dental work, drugs, viral illness or even menstruation and stress. Test for C1 esterase inhibitor deficiency/activity and complement levels. **Treatment:** ☠ Adrenaline, hydrocortisone and antihistamines are ineffective ☠. Acute

Rx requires urgent administration of C1 esterase inhibitor, either purified from human plasma (BERINERT, CINRYZE), or as recombinant conestat alpha (RUCONEST) or icatibant (FIRAZYR). Tranexamic acid 500 mg bd–tds po[SPC] or danazol 100–200 mg tds po (unlicensed indication and not in elderly or children[SPC]) can be used for prophylaxis several days before and after a planned procedure (e.g. surgery or dental work).

BRONCHIECTASIS EXACERBATION

Diagnosed clinically. **Clues include:** Sudden ↑SOB, lethargy, ↑T°, ↑cough, chest pain, haemoptysis, ↑ sputum viscosity or change in colour, wheeze, RR > 25/min, HR >110 or ↑CRP. **Emergency Rx** is the same as for COPD (page 241). However, reserve bronchodilators (salbutamol ± ipratropium ± aminophylline) and prednisolone for patients with signs of ↑airflow obstruction (e.g. wheeze or ↓FEV$_1$). Bronchiectasis patients can also retain CO$_2$ (prevention and Rx as per COPD). Choice of antibiotics depends on previously demonstrated colonising organism (e.g. PSEUDOMONAS) and the severity of exacerbation (po or iv). Antibiotics often continued for 2 wks (± ≥ 2 days) after sputum has cleared[NICE]. For antibiotic choices refer to Table 2.2.

CARBON MONOXIDE POISONING

Colourless, odourless gas formed from carbon burning with limited O$_2$. Acute inhalation can cause death. This can be accidental (e.g. faulty heating systems) or non-accidental (e.g. suicide with car exhaust fumes). Chronic low-grade inhalation can present non-specifically; suspect if several family members with similar symptoms. **Clues:** nausea, headache, malaise, unsteadiness, ↓GCS, seizures, cardiac ischaemia and 'cherry red' colour.

  Carbon monoxide (CO) binds avidly to haemoglobin (Hb) to form carboxyhaemoglobin (COHb). COHb → ↓ transportation and release of O$_2$ by Hb at the tissues. COHb can be measured in a heparinised venous sample. Normal levels are < 3% for non-smokers, or as high as 15% in smokers.

5.6.1 Important

COHb has similar absorption spectra to oxyhaemoglobin: pulse oximetry will be normal.

Arterial PO_2 levels may be normal.

MANAGEMENT
High flow O_2 (± CPAP or intubation) displaces CO from COHb. This allows ↑elimination from the body and ↑O_2 delivery to tissues. **Hyperbaric O_2** occasionally used.

COPD EXACERBATION

COPD exacerbations are diagnosed clinically. **Clues:** sudden ↑SOB, ↑cough, purulent discoloured sputum, wheeze, RR > 25/min, HR > 110 in a patient with emphysema, chronic bronchitis ± 'asthma'. Where possible, obtain a brief history early in the assessment. This helps guide Rx and escalation decisions, e.g. severity of underlying COPD, functional status/exercise tolerance. **NB:** *not all exacerbations require hospital admission → consider home Rx if appropriate with prednisolone 30 mg po od ± doxycycline 200 mg od po.*

EMERGENCY MANAGEMENT
Start Rx prior to investigations:

1. Sit patient upright
2. Attach O_2 sats probe (+ cardiac leads and BP cuff)
3. Administer 28% controlled O_2 through venturi mask. ☠ Beware CO_2 retention (discussed earlier)! ☠

5.7.1 CO_2 retention and O_2 therapy

☠ Beware CO_2 retention is all COPD patients ☠

Best prevented using the following target O_2 saturations:

- If known 'CO_2 retainer' → target 88–92%
- If *not* known 'CO_2 retainer' or ↔ CO_2 → target ≥ 94%

If O_2 sats < target → ↑FiO_2 cautiously and perform ABG to ensure not ↑CO_2/↓pH **Always prescribe O_2 on drug chart and state target O_2 sats.**

4. Salbutamol 2.5–5 mg via air-driven neb if possible (repeat every 15 min; > hourly seldom required)
5. Ipratropium 0.5 mg via air-driven neb if possible (repeat up to every 4–6 h if unwell)
6. Prednisolone 30 po od (usually 5–7 days). Hydrocortisone 100–200 mg qds iv can be given if unable to swallow or retain tablets (prednisolone as effective)
7. Doxycycline 200 mg od po (first dose) then 100 mg od po for total 5 days (first line) or amoxicillin/co-amoxiclav (usual second line), if features of infection (e.g ↑ing sputum volume or ↑ing purulence, ↑WCC/CRP)
8. Consider need for investigations, e.g. ABG, blood tests and CXR (exclude infection and pneumothorax).

In patients with severe exacerbations or those failing to improve, consider the following:

1. **Aminophylline ivi:** See Mx of asthma (page 136) for details.
2. **Ventilation:** Non-invasive first: NIV (BIPAP) for type 2 respiratory failure (↑PCO_2/↓pH) or CPAP for type 1 respiratory failure (↓PaO_2 with ↔ $PaCO_2$). Intubation and mechanical ventilation might be appropriate for some patients; decision can be difficult and should be discussed with the patient's consultant ± ITU.

3. **Doxapram:** If NIV not available (rarely used since the introduction of NIV). Use 1.5–4 mg/min ivi adjusted according to response. Seek senior advice and/or ITU involved.

5.7.2 Tips

- Discontinue inhalers if using regular nebs/prednisolone, but ensure reinitiated at discharge
- Exacerbations are perfect opportunities to review medication and inhaler technique
- Consider risk/benefit of continuing ICS if recurrent pneumonia
- Mobilise early to prevent deconditioning and muscle wasting
- Advise smoking cessation and offer Rx to current smokers
- Assess nutrition and need for supplementation
- Do *not* assess for LTOT *or* record spirometry during or immediately after an exacerbation (there may be exceptions)

CYSTIC FIBROSIS EXACERBATION

CF exacerbations are diagnosed clinically. **Clues include:** ↑cough, ↑ sputum viscosity or change in colour, ↑SOB, lethargy, fever (rare in CF), chest pain, haemoptysis, wheeze, weight loss, ↑CRP or ↓FEV$_1$ (± other features). Rx can be at home (even if iv antibiotics required) or in hospital. It may be appropriate to initially assess in an emergency clinic slot or on a day case unit. **NB:** not all exacerbations require CXR and blood tests, but they should be covered with appropriate antibiotics. Sputum MC&S or a cough swab should be sent (ideally prior to commencing antibiotics) (Box 5.8.1). It is important that all other CF Rx is continued with particular attention to glycaemic control, nutrition and chest physiotherapy.

5.8.1 Antibiotics in CF exacerbations

- Choice depends on colonising organism (most often *PSEUDOMONAS* in adults) *and* previous clinical response

- Follow local guidelines ± discuss with patient's consultant at earliest opportunity
- Please see page 83 for more details and alternatives

Typical regimen for Pseudomonal exacerbation:

- *Mild exacerbation:* Ciprofloxacin 750 mg bd po for 2 wks
- *Severe exacerbation:* Ceftazidime 2 g tds iv + tobramycin 7 mg/kg od iv for 2 wks

HAEMOPTYSIS

Small volume haemoptysis is common and a non-specific feature of many respiratory conditions. In practice the usual differential diagnosis is malignancy, bronchiectasis, infection/pneumonia, MTB and pulmonary embolism. In 1/3rd of patients, no cause is found. Investigations are tailored to the likely underlying cause, usually including a CT thorax and bronchoscopy.

Massive haemoptysis (> 100 mL/24 hours) is rare, but life-threatening (> 50% mortality). Usually encountered in patients with known lung conditions (e.g. CF, bronchiectasis or tumours).

☠ Massive haemoptysis arises from bronchial artery bleeding (i.e. systemic circulation under high pressure). immediate action + senior/ITU support is usually required. ☠

EMERGENCY MANAGEMENT OF MASSIVE HAEMOPTYSIS

Palliative Rx may be more appropriate to alleviate distress (page 114). Immediate life-saving Rx should be started before any investigations:

1. Protect airway (intubation if required/appropriate; consider double lumen endotracheal tube to isolate bleeding lung).
2. Between 40–60% FiO_2 through high-flow mask, e.g. Hudson mask. ☠ Beware ↑CO_2 with chronic lung conditions! ☠
3. Attach O_2 sats monitor (+ cardiac leads and BP cuff).

4. Protect unaffected lung by lying patient onto bleeding side (use CXR, previous CT or history to identify bleeding lung; patient can often tell from 'gurgling' sensation).

5. Insert large bore iv or central venous access; send blood for G&S and clotting.

6. Fluid resuscitate if required. However, permissive hypotension is advocated to slow the rate of bleeding (e.g. only treat to raise BP if sBP < 90 mmHg). If BP allows, administer GTN sl or ivi (50 mg in 50 mL sodium chloride 0.9% at initial rate 1 mg/h, adjusted according to response).

7. Nebulised adrenaline (use 1 mL of 1:1000 with 4 mL sodium chloride 0.9%).

8. Administer tranexamic acid po or iv (500 mg–1 g).

9. Consider terlipressin 2 mg iv (unlicensed indication).

10. Reverse any clotting abnormality (e.g. vitamin K for prolonged prothrombin time in CF or with warfarin).

11. Broad spectrum antibiotics iv (pulmonary blood is a good medium for bacterial growth).

Further management options include:

1. **Rigid bronchoscopy (intubated patient under GA):** Isolate and tamponade the bleeding site with a balloon. **NB:** *there is no role for flexible bronchoscopy in acute massive haemoptysis.*

2. **Bronchial artery angiography and embolization:** Attempted by interventional radiologists in some centres. The bleeding site can be difficult to ascertain/isolate. Risks inc. spinal artery (paraplegia) or systemic artery embolisation. Severe chest pain is a common side effect.

3. **Surgery:** Resection of bleeding lobe if all other measures fail.

ONCOLOGY EMERGENCIES

SUPERIOR VENA CAVAL OBSTRUCTION (SVCO)

Medical emergency: Obstructed flow within the SVC can result from external compression by tumour or lymph nodes, direct tumour invasion and/or venous thrombosis. Most cases (> 95%)

are secondary to lung cancer or lymphoma. Other malignant causes include thymoma and mediastinal tumours (primary/secondary). Benign causes include granulomatous disease, goitre, CVP lines, Port-a-Caths and pacemaker wires. **Diagnosis:** often presents with classical features (see Box 5.10.1) in a patient with known malignancy and is confirmed on CT imaging. SVCO often means surgical resection of the lung cancer is not possible.

5.10.1 Clinical features of SVCO

- Headache (often worse on bending forwards)
- Syncope or dizziness ($\downarrow$venous return)
- Associated features (e.g. SOB, cough, haemoptysis, hoarse voice, dysphagia)
- Facial and upper body oedema
- Facial plethora/cyanotic appearance
- Venous distension of face and upper body (often chest)

Management
Best practice: Histological confirmation before treatment. Chemotherapy, radiotherapy and even steroids can influence histology. Do *not* delay; expedite biopsy if cause of SVCO unknown.
General measures: Sit patient upright, O_2, analgesia and steroids to reduce oedema, e.g. dexamethasone 8 mg bd po, avoiding evening doses (disturb sleep). Further Rx depends on the underlying disease. Broadly SCLC or lymphoma $\rightarrow$ chemotherapy *and* NCSL $\rightarrow$ radiotherapy $\pm$ SVC stent insertion.

SPINAL CORD COMPRESSION
Prompt Rx required to prevent irreversible paraplegia $\pm$ loss of bowel or bladder function. ☠ **Have a low threshold for investigating back pain in a patient with known cancer!** ☠ Can result from direct spread of a vertebral metastasis (most common), external cord compression, vertebral artery compromise or

metastasis within the cord. **Clues:** back pain (not always!), weak legs with loss of sensation and upper motor neurone signs, loss of bowel or bladder function (constipation, urinary retention or incontinence; usually late signs) and saddle sensory loss with ↓anal tone (cauda equina). **Investigation:** urgent MRI spine.

Management

Start high-dose steroids when clinically suspected, e.g. dexamethasone 8 mg iv bd. Catheterise, start DVT prophylaxis (LMWH) and use a pressure-relieving mattress. Always discuss with patient's oncologist ± neurosurgeon. Options include radiotherapy to single/multiple sites or surgical decompression, reconstruction and stabilisation.

HYPERCALCAEMIA

Serum Ca^{2+} > 2.65 mmol/L; Ca^{2+} > 3 mmol/L is usually symptomatic, and Ca^{2+} > 3.25 mmol/L usually secondary to malignancy. **NB:** ↑PTH in hyperparathyroidism but ↓PTH in malignancy. Typical features include confusion, weakness, constipation, abdominal pain, nausea, renal failure and ↓QTc.

Management

Commence treatment if symptomatic *or* Ca^{2+} > 3.5 mmol/L:

1. Normal saline (0.9%) ivi 1 L 4–6 hrly
2. If no improvement consider furosemide (loop diuretic; never use thiazides which ↑ Ca^{2+}), bisphosphonates (e.g. disodium pamidronate single infusion usually[SPC] 15–60 mg ivi over 2 h, or as multiple infusions in divided doses over 2–4 days; max. 90 mg per treatment course) or corticosteroids.

SYNDROME OF INAPPROPRIATE SECRETION OF ANTIDIURETIC HORMONE (SIADH)

Inappropriate production of antidiuretic hormone (ADH) →↑water retention and a hypo-osmolar state: ↓Na^+, urine osmolality > 100 mosmol/kg and urine Na^+ > 40 mmol/L. Respiratory causes include SCLC and pneumonia.

Management

Fluid restriction (0.5–1 L/d) ± demeclocycline usually 450 mg bd po initially and for maintenance[BNF].

OTHERS

Haemoptysis (page 244) and upper airway obstruction (page 269).

PULMONARY EMBOLISM

Very common! Have a low index of suspicion in patients with risk factors or compatible clinical presentation. **Important symptoms:** SOB (73%), chest pain (66% – *not* always pleuritic), cough (37%), apprehension, sweating, haemoptysis and syncope. ☠ PE can be asymptomatic and only detected incidentally. ☠ **Important signs:** ↑RR > 20/min (70%), crepitations (51%), ↑PR (30%) and low grade ↑T°. ☠ **NB:** NOT all patients with PE (inc even larger PE) are hypoxic at rest; some may only desaturate on mobilisation and some may not be hypoxic at all! ☠

5.11.1 Initial management of PE

Consider the following before arranging investigations:

High flow O_2: If hypoxic. ☠ Beware COPD and type 2 respiratory failure. ☠

Analgesia: If pain or distress, try paracetamol/ibuprofen 1st; consider opiates ONLY if severe or no response (☠ respiratory depression ☠).

Fluids (± inotropes): If haemodynamic compromise (supports circulation by maintaining RV filling) and consider early thrombolysis (discussed hereunder).

LMWH, e.g. enoxaparin or dalteparin: Start weight-adjusted sc dose once PE is suspected (may be prior to CTPA).

Thrombolysis alteplase: May be indicated prior to investigation in those with a high-clinical probability of acute PE and haemodynamic instability. This requires senior clinical judgement and in practice, there may *not*

---

be time for a CTPA or Echo. ☠ Delay in reperfusion could precipitate a cardiac arrest. Ensure alternative reasonable diagnoses are excluded. ☠

Clinical investigations that may provide important clues:

ECG: Sinus tachycardia most common; also AF, RAD, RBBB, anterior T wave $\downarrow$ and $S_1Q_3T_3$ (rare and neither sensitive nor specific).
ABG: Frequently normal, but may show $\downarrow PO_2$ (or $\uparrow$ A-a gradient) $\pm$ $\downarrow PCO_2$ (hyperventilation).
CXR: Frequently normal; may show small effusions, infiltrates, atelectasis or the cause of PE (e.g. lung cancer). 'Westermark's' sign (oligaemia), 'Palla's' sign (abrupt ending pulmonary artery) and 'Hampton's hump' (wedge-shaped pulmonary infarction) are rare and/or subtle.
D-dimer: Fibrin degradation product; $\uparrow$after a blood clot is degraded by fibrinolysis. Sensitive but not specific. ☠ Only use in conjunction with a pre-test clinical probability score (discussed hereunder). ☠
Troponin: May be $\uparrow$ and is a marker of RV strain.

Common diagnostic investigations:

CT Pulmonary Angiogram (CTPA): Test of choice. Will show filling defects in pulmonary vasculature; may identify signs of RV compromise (e.g. $\uparrow$RV size, interventricular septal bowing, $\uparrow$PA).
VQ Scan: Generally reserved for younger patients (esp female). Will show ventilation-perfusion mismatches: A high-probability scan defined as showing ≥ 2 unmatched segmental perfusion defects (PIOPED criteria). Performing a perfusion scan only may be acceptable when the chest X-ray is normal (any perfusion defect considered to be a mismatch).
VQ SPECT: Single photon emission CT ventilation/perfusion imaging is increasingly available and has replaced VQ scans in many hospital trusts.
Echocardiography: $\uparrow$use for haemodynamically unstable patients. Larger acute PE $\rightarrow$ $\uparrow$RV pressure and dysfunction, detectable on Echo. May show mobile right heart thrombi.

ASSESSMENT OF ACUTE PE

The initial assessment of any suspected acute PE should focus on assessing PE severity according to mortality risk. Those at greatest risk of death are hypotensive (systolic BP < 90 mmHg) or have evidence of shock. They should be considered for early reperfusion therapy (e.g. systemic thrombolysis). A detailed assessment of mortality risk combines several key indicators, including clinical features, PE severity index (PESI) or simplified PESI scoring (Figure 5.1), CTPA ± echo features and troponin values[ESC] (Table 5.1). According to ESC guidance, suspected acute PE can be classified as 'High risk',

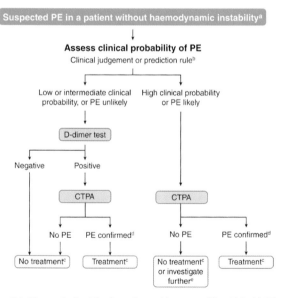

Figure 5.1 Diagnostic algorithm for patients with suspected 'not high-risk PE' (i.e. absence of shock or hypotension). (Adapted from ESC Guidelines [2019]).

Table 5.1 Classification of PE severity and mortality risk

Early mortality risk		Indicators of risk			
		Haemodynamic instability[a]	Clinical parameters of PE severity and/or comorbidity: PESI class III–V or sPESI ≥1	RV dysfunction on TTE or CTPA[b]	Elevated cardiac troponin levels[c]
High		+	(+)[d]	+	(+)[d]
Intermediate	Intermediate-high	–	+[e]	+	+
	Intermediate-low	–	+[e]	One (or none) positive	
Low		–	–	Assessment optional; if assessed, negative	

BP: blood pressure; CTPA: computed tomography pulmonary angiography; H-FABP: heart-type fatty acid-binding protein; NT-proBNP: N-terminal pro B-type natriuretic peptide; PE: pulmonary embolism; PESI: Pulmonary Embolism Severity Index; RV: right ventricular; sPESI: simplified Pulmonary Embolism Severity Index; TTE: transthoracic echocardiogram. [a]One of the following clinical presentations (table 4): cardiac arrest, obstructive shock (systolic BP <90 mmHg or vasopressors required to achieve a BP ≥90 mmHg despite an adequate filling status, in combination with end-organ hypoperfusion), or persistent hypotension (systolic BP <90 mmHg or a systolic BP drop ≥40 mmHg for >15 min, not caused by new-onset arrhythmia, hypovolaemia, or sepsis). [b]Prognostically relevant imaging (TTE or CTPA) findings in patients with acute PE, and the corresponding cut-off levels, are graphically presented in figure 3, and their prognostic value is summarized in table 3. [c]Elevation of further laboratory biomarkers, such as NT-proBNP ≥600 ng/L, H-FABP ≥6 ng/mL, or copeptin ≥24 pmol/ L, may provide additional prognostic information. These markers have been validated in cohort studies but they have not yet been used to guide treatment decisions in randomized controlled trials. [d]Haemodynamic instability, combined with PE confirmation on CTPA and/or evidence of RV dysfunction on TTE, is sufficient to classify a patient into the high-risk PE category. In these cases, neither calculation of the PESI nor measurement of troponins or other cardiac biomarkers is necessary. [e]Signs of RV dysfunction on TTE (or CTPA) or elevated cardiac biomarker levels may be present, despite a calculated PESI of I–II or an sPESI of 0 [234]. Until the implications of such discrepancies for the management of PE are fully understood, these patients should be classified into the intermediate-risk category.

European Society of Cardiology Guidelines 2019.

'Intermediate-high risk', 'Intermediate-low risk' and 'low risk'. Suggested investigations and Rx depend on this risk assessment (as discussed hereunder).

'High-risk' acute PE

🔔 Suspected high-risk PE is immediately life-threatening (analogous to 'Massive PE')! 🔔 Table 5.2. Do NOT delay investigations or manage on ambulatory care pathways (also true if clinical signs or investigations suggest RV strain but no shock/↓BP). Patients are haemodynamically unstable or arrested, and reperfusion (e.g. thrombolysis) prior to confirming PE on CTPA/echo may be preferable (see Box). Otherwise, if appropriate, immediately anticoagulate patient (LMWH or UFH) and urgently arrange CTPA/Echo to confirm PE (and exclude alternative diagnoses) prior to reperfusion. Options for reperfusion are (dependent on local guidance and availability):

- **Systemic thrombolysis:** Most commonly with alteplase. Restores perfusion more rapidly than UFH/LMWH alone and is potentially life-saving! ALWAYS perform an individual 'risk vs. benefit' assessment, consider relative and absolute

Table 5.2 PESI and sPESI risk stratification

	PESI	sPESI
Age	+ *Age (years)*	+ *1 (Age > 80 years)*
Male sex	+ 10	–
Cancer	+ 30	+1
Chronic heart failure	+ 10	+1
Chronic pulmonary disease	+ 10	
PR ≥ 110 bpm	+ 20	+1
sBP < 100 mmHg	+ 30	+1
RR > 30 breaths/min	+ 20	–
Temperature < 36°C	+ 20	–
Confusion	+ 60	
Arterial oxyhaemoglobin saturation < 90%	+ 20	+ 1 point

Risk stratification

≤ 65 points: Class I (0–1.6% 30-day mortality = very low) 66–85 points: Class II (1.7–3.5% 30-day mortality = low) 86–105 points: Class III (3.2–7.1% 30-day mortality = moderate) 106–125 points: Class IV (4.0–11.4% 30-day mortality = high) >125 points: Class V (10.0–24.5% 30-day mortality = very high)	**0 points:** 30-day mortality = 1.0% **≥1 point:** 30-day mortality = 10.9%

contraindications to thrombolysis. Alternative Rx (discussed hereunder) are available in some centres and useful when thrombolysis is contraindicated or the risk of bleeding is high.

- **Half-dose thrombolysis:** Used in some centres as ↓bleeding risk.
- **Surgical embolectomy:** Rarely performed but consider if thrombolysis is contraindicated or has failed for 'high risk'/'intermediate-high risk' patients; seek urgent cardiothoracic opinion.
- **Catheter-directed therapy:** Administers localised thrombolysis or achieves embolectomy by mechanical disruption or suction.

For specific treatments please refer to anticoagulation (page 148) and thrombolysis (page 188). **Vena cava filters** are occasionally used (inserted under radiology-guidance) in acute high-risk PE, where a second 'episode' might be fatal. Also used when anticoagulation is absolutely contraindicated or when recurrent PE occurs despite optimum anticoagulation.

'Not High-Risk' acute PE

For patients with suspected 'not high-risk' acute PE (i.e. 'Intermediate risk' and 'Low risk'; NO signs of shock or ↓BP), first stratify by clinical probability of PE. Several probability assessments exist. A two-tier Wells score is easy to apply. It classifies the patient as 'PE likely' or 'PE unlikely' (Table 5.3). It determines the need for D-dimer blood testing (Figure 5.2): a negative D-dimer can reliably exclude PE after a 'PE unlikely' risk assessment (low probability), so avoiding the need for CTPA. ☠ D-dimers should NOT be performed (or results applied) in the event of a 'PE likely' (high probability) assessment, as a -ve result can NOT reliably exclude PE! ☠

Management of 'Not High-Risk' acute PE:

For most cases of 'intermediate-' and 'low'-risk acute PE (i.e. without/↓BP) anticoagulation (without reperfusion) is adequate, i.e. LMWH followed by warfarin, or DOAC. Start LMWH (weight-adjusted dose) before starting warfarin, or use DOAC. Treatment can be commenced before the confirmation of PE. 'Intermediate risk' patients SHOULD be admitted and NOT managed on

Table 5.3 Two-tier Wells score (example of a simple clinical probability assessment)

Clinical feature	Points
Clinical signs and symptoms of DVT (minimum of leg swelling and pain on palpation of deep veins)	3
Alternative diagnosis less likely than PE	3
Heart rate > 100 bpm	1.5
Immobilisation > 3 days or surgery in last 4 wks	1.5
Previous DVT/PE	1.5
Haemoptysis	1
Malignancy (on Rx, Rx in last 6 months or palliative)	1
Clinical probability score	
'PE Likely'	> 4 points
'PE Unlikely'	≤ 4 points

ambulatory pathways, whereas low-risk patients may be safely discharged early/managed on ambulatory pathways (where practical/supported by local guidelines)^{ESC}. CLOSELY monitor 'intermediate-high risk' patients for circulatory decompensation and consider **early rescue reperfusion** if this develops (i.e. full dose thrombolysis, half-dose thrombolysis, surgical embolectomy or catheter-directed Rx). It is reasonable to maintain such patients on LMWH during this period of observation. Routine primary reperfusion with systemic thrombolysis is NOT currently recommended for 'intermediate-high risk' patients (concerns over risk of bleeding and lack of clear evidence for benefit)^{ESC}.

Further Top Tips

- ☠ Warfarin is teratogenic and should NOT be used in pregnancy! ☠ Use LMWH sc until ≥6 wks after delivery.
- Long-term LMWH (not warfarin) is Rx of choice for patients with malignancy.
- When recent/impending surgery, or if rapid reversal is anticipated, consider heparin.

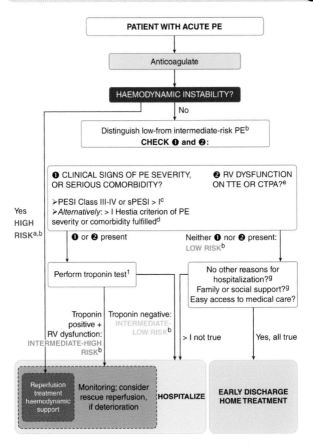

Figure 5.2 Management of acute PE according to risk (Adapted from ESC Guidelines [2019]).

- Plan follow-up at discharge, esp for 'unprovoked' PE (no clear aetiology; investigations for cancer may be warranted) and larger PE (ensure clot resolution and follow-up for possible 2° pulmonary hypertension).

PNEUMONIA

Acute lower respiratory tract infection (LRTI) with new radiographic shadowing (consolidation). Usually bacterial, occasionally viral. Distinguish from non-pneumonic LRTI (e.g. acute bronchitis), which is often viral (antibiotics frequently *not* required). Pneumonia can be community-acquired (CAP), hospital-acquired (HAP), ventilator-associated (VAP) or caused by aspiration. Complications include abscess formation, cavitation and effusion (parapneumonic/empyema).

EMERGENCY MANAGEMENT OF PNEUMONIA

Diagnosis is clinical: Symptoms, signs and new CXR changes. Clues: ↑T°, SOB, cough, sputum, confusion, malaise, anorexia, haemoptysis, ↑RR, shock, hypoxia, localising signs of consolidation and pleural rub. Obtain brief history early in assessment to help identify risk factors for specific organisms and guide further Rx, e.g. need for admission (CURB-65) or appropriateness of intubation if deterioration, i.e. comorbidity, functional status/exercise tolerance.

Approach to emergency management:

1. Sit patient upright
2. Attach O_2 sats monitor (+ cardiac leads and BP cuff)
3. Administer O_2, ensure O_2 sats ≥ 94% (☠ controlled O_2 with target sats 88–92% if type 2 respiratory failure ☠)
4. ABG if hypoxia
5. Rx hypotension and shock as necessary (IV fluids ± catheter)
6. Consider other Rx (e.g. 2.5–5 mg salbutamol neb if wheezy)

7. Consider investigations – bloods, CXR, sputum/blood cultures, pneumonia serology
8. Commence antibiotics early (IV and within 1 h if any signs of sepsis) – discussed hereunder
9. Consider VTE prophylaxis, nutritional support (esp if prolonged illness suspected) and chest physiotherapy (airway clearance)
10. Early ITU referral, esp if severe CAP, $PO_2 < 8$ kPa despite high-flow O_2, tiring patient (e.g. $\uparrow CO_2$), $\downarrow$ consciousness level or signs of persistent shock despite adequate iv fluids ($\downarrow$pH, $\uparrow$lactate or $\downarrow$ urine output)

Community-acquired pneumonia (CAP)

Common infection acquired in the community. Smokers, alcoholics, diabetics, the immunocompromised, patients with chronic lung conditions and nursing home residents are more susceptible. Severity and prognosis can be assessed using the CURB-65 score (discussed hereunder) (Box 5.12.1). Other poor prognostic factors include: respiratory failure ($PaO_2 < 8$ kPa), albumin < 35 g/L, WCC < 20 or $< 4 \times 10^9$/L, bilateral or multilobar consolidation, bacteraemia (cultures) and comorbid conditions (e.g. CCF or diabetes). **Follow-up:** always arrange CXR at around 6 wks to ensure radiological resolution (☠ to look for underlying condition, e.g. cancer ☠). Consider CT and bronchoscopy if inadequate resolution of CAP. **NB:** legionella, pneumococcal and extensive pneumonia may resolve more slowly.

5.12.1 Severity assessment of CAP in hospital[1]

'CURB 65' score – *1 point each for:*
   Confusion: MTS[2] $\leq$ 8/10 or *new* disorientation in time, place or person
   Urea > 7 mmol/L
   Respiratory rate $\geq$ 30/min
   BP$\downarrow$: Systolic < 90 mmHg **or** diastolic $\leq$ 60 mmHg
   65: Age $\geq$ 65 yr

<2: Non-severe; likely to be suitable for home treatment.

=2: Moderate with *increased* risk of death; consider admission (or hospital supervised outpatient care) using clinical judgement.

≥2: Severe with *high* risk of death; admit and consider HDU/ITU (esp if ≥4).

---

[1] For assessment in the community use *'CRB 65'*, no need for blood test: 0 = likely to be suitable for home treatment; 1–2 = consider hospital referral; 3–4 = urgent hospital admission.

[2] MTS = Mental Test Score; see for details.

Adapted with permission of BMJ Publishing Group from BTS guidelines. *Thorax* 2001; 56 (suppl IV) and 2009 update.

Treatment

Non-severe: Amoxicillin 500 mg–1 g tds po ± clarithromycin 500 mg bd po (if admitted for clinical reasons). Patients managed in community should receive Rx for 7 days.

Severe: Co-amoxiclav 1.2 g tds iv + clarithromycin 500 mg bd iv ± flucloxacillin 1 g qds iv, if *S. aureus* (Hx or epidemic of flu) ± rifampicin 600 mg bd po/iv if *Legionella* (do urinary Ag test). Consider IV → po Rx as soon as patient clinically improves and afebrile for 24 h. Patients admitted to hospital should receive 7–10 days Rx, longer if clinically appropriate, e.g. empyema.

Failure to improve: Ensure correct diagnosis (e.g. exclude PE, LVF, cancer, cryptogenic organising pneumonia) and look for pneumonia complications (e.g. empyema). Consider co-amoxiclav → TAZOCIN (piperacillin + tazobactam).

- If risk factors, consider Rx for aspiration or TB (AAFB confirmation preferred prior to commencing).
- If penicillin hypersensitivity, use clarithromycin only.

Clarithromycin is better tolerated than erythromycin (↓GI upset); consult local protocol to check preference.

5.12.2 Microbiology of CAP (UK adults)

48% ***Streptococcus pneumoniae ('pneumococcus'):*** Esp in winter or overcrowding, e.g. shelters/prison.

23% ***Viruses:*** Influenza (A ≫ B), RSV, rhinoviruses, adenoviruses.

15% ***Chlamydia psittaci:*** Esp. from animals, but only 20% from birds (less commonly *Chlamydia pneumoniae*, esp if long-term Hx and headache).

7% ***Haemophilus influenzae.***

3% ***Mycoplasma pneumoniae:*** ↑s during 4-yrly epidemics.

3% ***Legionella pneumophila:*** ↑d if recent travel (esp Turkey, Spain).

2% ***Moraxella catarrhalis:*** ↑d in elderly.

1.5% ***Staphylococcus aureus:*** Mostly post-influenza ∴ ↑s in winter.

1.4% **Gram-negative infection:** Escherichia coli, *PSEUDOMONAS*, Klebsiella, Proteus, Serratia.

1.1% **Anaerobes:** E.g. Bacteroides, Fusobacterium.

0.7% ***Coxiella burnetii* (Q fever):** ↑s in April–June and in sheep farmers.

The causative pathogen is not identified in ≥ 20% of cases and ≈ 25% are of mixed aetiology. Avoid the term "atypical pathogen" (refers to *Mycoplasma, Chlamydia, Coxiella, Legionella*) as there is no characteristic clinical presentation for the pneumonia they cause.

- **Microbiological investigations: *Non-severe*** – no microbiological investigation routinely required;
- ***Moderate & Severe*** – blood culture, sputum MC&S, pneumococcal urine antigen, legionella urine antigen (+ sputum for MC&S and immunofluorescence) and PCR/serology for viral causes or mycoplasma.

Adapted with permission of BMJ Publishing Group from Lim WS, *et al.* Thorax 2001; **56**: 296–301.

Hospital-acquired pneumonia (HAP)

LRTI associated with consolidation ≥ 72 h after hospital admission. Often results from aspiration of colonised URT secretions, haematogenous spread of microorganisms or inhalation of bacteria.

Treatment

Non-severe: Co-amoxiclav 625 mg tds po.
Severe (or if NBM): Co-amoxiclav 1.2 g tds iv *or* TAZOCIN (piperacillin + tazobactam) 4.5 g tds iv if *PSEUDOMONAS* suspected. Meropenem 1 g tds iv if penicillin allergy (☠ NEVER prescribe if history of anaphylactic or accelerated allergic reaction – discuss alternatives with microbiologist). ☠ Consider co-therapy with gentamicin if septic shock or failure to improve.
MRSA: Teicoplanin/vancomycin if colonisation or demonstrated on respiratory MC&S.

5.12.3 Microbiology of HAP

Simple: (within 7 days of admission): *H. influenzae,*
S. pneumoniae, S. aureus, Gram-negative organisms.
Complicated*: Gram-negative organisms (esp *P. aeruginosa*),
Acinetobacter, MRSA.
Anaerobic**: *Bacteroides, Fusobacterium.*

Special situations:

1 Head trauma, coma, DM, RF: Consider *S. aureus.*
2 Mini-epidemics in hospitals: Consider *Legionella.*

* > 7 days after admission, recent multiple antibiotics or complex medical Hx (e.g. recent
ITU/recurrent admissions or severe comorbidity).
**Esp if risk of aspiration, recent abdominal surgery, bronchial obstruction/poor
dentition.

Reproduced with permission from Hammersmith Hospitals NHS Trust Clinical Management
Guidelines & Formulary 2001.

Aspiration pneumonia

Pneumonia following aspiration of foreign material into the LRT, usually oropharyngeal or gastric contents. Insult is a combination of chemical pneumonitis (intense inflammatory reaction), bacterial infection (commonly anaerobes) and mechanical obstruction (e.g. from gastric contents).

Treatment: As for CAP or HAP + metronidazole 500 mg tds iv or 400 mg tds po.

Ventilator-associated pneumonia

Pneumonia in mechanically ventilated patient $\geq$ 48 h after intubation. Typically a consequence of bacterial contamination of LRT from aspiration not prevented by cuffed endotracheal tubes or tracheostomy.

Treatment: Always consult local policies ± microbiologist. Drug-resistant organisms are common.

Cavitating pneumonia

Complication of a severe-necrotising pneumonia. Also consider TB, septic emboli and non-infectious causes (e.g. malignancy).

Treatment: Co-amoxiclav 1.2 g tds iv. Consider flucloxacillin 1 g qds iv (if *S. aureus* suspected) or vancomycin iv + rifampicin po (if MRSA suspected/confirmed).

5.12.4 Cavity

> Cancer
> Autoimmune (e.g. Wegener's)
> Vascular (e.g. septic pulmonary emboli)
> Infection (Think 'TANKS')
> Trauma (e.g. pneumatocoeles)
> Youth (e.g. bronchogenic cyst or pulmonary sequestration)
>
> **"TANKS" Cause Cavitation**
>
> *T*B, *Aspergillus*, *Nocardia*, *Klebsiella*, *S. aureus*
> (and *PSEUDOMONAS*)

PNEUMOTHORAX

Air in the pleural cavity occurring spontaneously or following trauma. This book covers spontaneous pneumothorax (PTx) in patients with normal lungs ('primary'; usually air leaking from an apical bleb in the 'classical' tall young thin man) or those with underlying lung disease ('secondary'). **Clues:** pleuritic chest pain, SOB (can be minimal in young patient with primary PTx), ↑PR, ↓chest expansion, ↑percussion resonance, ↓breath sounds, subcutaneous ('surgical') emphysema and hypoxic. ☠ There may be no signs, and PTx is only visible on CXR. ☠ The PTx can also act as a one-way valve to create a tension PTx (see Box).

5.13.1 Tension pneumothorax

☠ **Medical emergency.** ☠ Progressively ↑ pleural pressure → ↓venous return, mediastinal shift and cardiac arrest.

If suspected clinically:

- Never delay Rx or wait for a CXR!
- Immediate high-flow O_2
- Immediate needle decompression with wide-bore cannula inserted into 2nd intercostal space, mid-clavicular line on the side of the pneumothorax → a 'hiss' from the pleural space is diagnostic
- Insert chest drain immediately after (leaving cannula in-situ until drain is bubbling)

Imaging: CXR is diagnostic in most cases. Measure the rim of PTx at the level of the hilum: > 2 cm = large (approximately 50% volume loss), < 2 cm = small. Small PTx might require lateral decubitus or expiratory CXR. CT can also help identify small PTx and distinguish bulla from PTx, identify any underlying lung conditions or apical blebs.

Treatment of spontaneous PTx: There are several management options. Always follow local guidelines or the BTS algorithm below.

5.13.2 Top practical tips for the management of spontaneous pneumothorax

Consult BTS guidelines for the Rx of spontaneous PTx.

Pleural procedures are too often attempted! Many PTx CAN be managed conservatively.

If attempting pleural aspiration, do *not* aspirate > 2 L; this is indicative of a large PTx, for which aspiration alone is unlikely to be successful.

Successful aspiration is defined as complete *or* near-complete lung re-expansion on CXR.

Delay a 'check' CXR for at least 1 h after aspiration, so as not to miss a slow air leak. Perform a second film later if not sure.

Beware pleural procedures in patients with apical/small) PTx! Ask yourself if they require any intervention at all (i.e. not symptomatic, or SOB not caused by PTx). If they do require intervention (e.g. small PTx has decompensated SOB in severe underlying lung disease) then consider the need for radiological guidance.

Small pleural drains (e.g. Seldinger 10–14 F) are often sufficient. Reserve larger bore drains for ↑air leaks, severe subcutaneous emphysema or ventilated patients (tube blockage may lead to tension PTx).

Drains are painful! Always use adequate lignocaine for insertion (± morphine or sedation IF SAFE!) and ensure adequate analgesia is prescribed afterwards: regular paracetamol + NSAID (e.g. ibuprofen) with opiate (e.g. codeine or oramorph) for break-through pain.

☠ Never clamp a bubbling chest drain! ☠ This will cause a tension PTx.

☠ Never start NIV with a PTx (may cause tension). ☠ Wait until a drain has been inserted.

If a drain stops swinging with respiration consider whether it is kinked, blocked (try normal saline flushes), accidentally clamped or has come out.

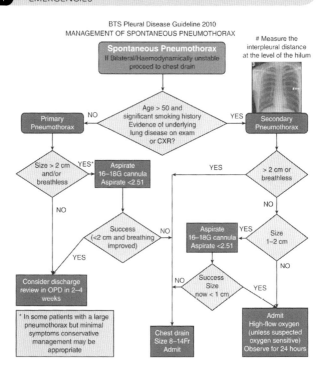

Figure 5.13.1 Management of spontaneous PTx. (BTS 2010 Pleural Disease Guideline).

Unless contraindicated (e.g. ↑PCO$_2$), all hospitalised patients should receive high-flow O$_2$ to aid PTx resolution.

Persistent air leaks: Some drains bubble > 48 h after insertion. Indicates that the air leak has failed to seal. Discuss with cardiothoracic team early: surgery may be required (discussed hereunder). *Other options include:* a 2nd chest drain, a larger bore drain or high volume-low pressure drain suction (only use purpose-made units available on chest ward; typically 3–5 kPa ≈ 30–50 cm H_2O). Some centres manage suitable patients with ambulatory chest drain systems.

Subcutaneous ('surgical') emphysema: Air tracks from the pleural space to below the SC tissue. Occurs with larger air leaks, a blocked chest drain or when the holes of the drain lie SC. Small amounts harmless. ☠ If severe → can compromise respiration. ☠ Check drain position and patency (i.e. swinging/bubbling and flushed). Discuss with cardiothoracics. Consider high-flow O_2 and insertion of a larger-bore drain ± suction.

Surgery: An apical bleb or air leak can be repaired by open thoracotomy or more commonly video-assisted thoracoscopic surgery (VATS). The pleural space can also be closed with abrasion, talc or partial pleurectomy. Surgery is reserved for patients with persistent air leaks, those with recurrent PTx (typically ipsilateral) or patients with risky professions (e.g. pilots or divers). In high-risk surgical candidates with recurrent PTx, consider talc pleurodesis via an intercostal drain.

Patient advice: Discuss smoking cessation, flying (after > 1 wk of documented PTx resolution) and diving (not until after definitive surgical procedure).

RESPIRATORY FAILURE

The respiratory system is responsible for effective gas exchange, i.e. oxygenation and CO_2 elimination. Respiratory failure (✖) results in hypoxaemia ($PO_2 < 8$ kPa) ± hypercapnia ($PCO_2 > 6.5$ kPa) (Box 5.14.1). It is defined as: (1) Type 1 or Type 2 (2) Acute (min, h, few days) or chronic (days to wks).

MANAGEMENT OF ACUTE TYPE 1 RESPIRATORY FAILURE

1. Administer high flow FiO_2 (via non-rebreathe mask) targeting O_2 sats > 92% ($PO_2 > 8$ kPa)
2. Treat underlying cause (e.g. diuretic for LVF)
3. If $PO_2 < 8$ kPa despite $FiO_2 \geq 60\%$ → consider mechanical ventilation, CPAP or high-flow nasal cannulae (e.g. Optiflow™)

5.14.1 Defining respiratory failure

TYPE 1 RESPIRATORY FAILURE (HYPOXAEMIC)

$PO_2 < 8$ kPa $\underline{\&} \leftrightarrow PCO_2$ (can be $\downarrow$ if hyperventilation)

Results from VQ mismatch

- Can be *'acute'* or *'chronic'* (often clinically compensated)
- *Causes include: Pneumonia, LVF, PE, COPD, asthma, bronchiectasis, ILD, pneumothorax, ARDS, pulmonary hypertension or obesity*

TYPE 2 RESPIRATORY FAILURE (HYPERCAPNIC)

$PO_2 < 8$kPa $\underline{\&}$ $PCO_2 > 6.5$ kPa

Results from alveolar hypoventilation

- Can be *'acute'* ($\uparrow PCO_2 \rightarrow \downarrow pH < 7.35$), *'chronic'* (renal compensation $\rightarrow \uparrow HCO_3 \rightarrow pH > 7.35$) or *'acute-on-chronic'/'decompensated chronic'* ($\uparrow HCO_3$ but $\rightarrow \downarrow pH < 7.35$)
- *Causes include: COPD, asthma, bronchiectasis, obesity, progression from type 1* ✖ *(tiring of respiratory muscles), sedatives, head injury, neuromuscular disease (e.g. diaphragmatic paralysis, poliomyelitis, MG, GBS) or kyphoscoliosis*

MANAGEMENT OF ACUTE TYPE 2 RESPIRATORY FAILURE

1. Administer controlled O_2 (via Venturi) targeting O_2 sats 88–92%
2. Treat underlying cause (e.g. bronchodilators for COPD)
3. Recheck ABG after 20–30 min:
   - If O_2 sats 88–92% and $PCO_2 \downarrow$ then continue Rx and controlled O_2
   - If $\uparrow PCO_2 \rightarrow$ consider mechanical ventilation or NIV (esp. if pH < 7.3)

Chronic ✖ (type 1 & 2) does not always require acute Rx (e.g. CPAP/NIV). Assess whether patient is decompensated.

SICKLE CELL DISEASE AND ACUTE CHEST SYNDROME

GENERAL POINTS

- Autosomal recessive
- Common in those from Africa (esp Equatorial), Middle East, central India and Nepal
- Characterised by production of abnormal ß globulin subunits of Hb (amino acid substitution of glutamine → valine). This forms HbS, rather than normal HbA
- In homozygotes, Hb electrophoresis → 80–99% HbS without HbA
- HbS polymerises (esp under $\downarrow O_2$) to create deformed and fragile RBCs (sickle)
- Sickled RBCs undergo chronic haemolysis ($\downarrow$Hb 60–90 g/L; $\uparrow$reticulocytes 10–20%) with vascular occlusion (micro) and tissue infarction
- Patients frequently experience 'crises' in response to cold, dehydration, infection or hypoxia
- Heterozygotes (30–40% HbS with 50% HbA) have sickle cell trait; largely asymptomatic but may sickle with extreme $\downarrow O_2$ (e.g. surgery)

5.15.1 Chronic pulmonary complications of sickle cell disease

- **Pneumonia:** More common in functionally asplenic (invasive pneumococcal, *Chlamydia pneumoniae*, *S. pneumoniae*, *H. influenzae*, *Mycoplasma*, *Legionella* and viral). May precipitate acute chest syndrome. Use prophylactic phenoxymethylpenicillin and vaccinate vs. *S. pneumoniae*.
- **Asthma:** More common but pathogenesis not fully understood. Standard Rx.
- **Nocturnal hypoxaemia and obstructive sleep apnoea:** Complex aetiology – tonsillar hypertrophy plays a role.

- **Pulmonary thromboembolic disease:** More common and may precipitate crisis including acute chest syndrome.
- **Sickle cell chronic lung disease:** Thought to be 2° to recurrent lung infarction $\pm$ infection (poorly understood). Mainly fibrotic (restrictive spirometry with HRCT findings).
- **Pulmonary hypertension:** Common. Rx as per idiopathic pulmonary hypertension

ACUTE CHEST SYNDROME

ALI which can rapidly progress to ARDS ($\approx$ 10–15% require mechanical ventilation). Typically acute onset $\uparrow T°$, cough, chest pain, SOB + new pulmonary infiltrate on CXR (consolidation) and hypoxia (O_2 sats < 94%, or > 3% below baseline). Often precipitated by infection, but bony crises (fat embolism), pulmonary infarction 2° to sequestration/PE, or hypoventilation during an acute crisis (atelectasis) can also play roles. ☠ **All patients with painful vaso-occlusion crises should be monitored closely for signs of acute chest syndrome.** ☠

Acute management

Contact haematology early!

1. **O_2:** High flow unless contraindicated; very low threshold for regular ABGs
2. **IV fluids:** But avoid over hydration (leaky pulmonary capillaries $\rightarrow \downarrow$ gas exchange)
3. **Broad-spectrum antibiotics:** Include a macrolide (e.g. Co-amoxiclav 1.2 g tds iv + clarithromycin 500 mg bd po/iv)
4. **Analgesia:** Vital to allow adequate inspiration and avoid atelectasis with further $\downarrow PO_2$ and sickling. Use NSAID $\pm$ opiates. ☠ Overnarcosis and hypoventilation ☠
5. **Nebulised bronchodilators:** Often helpful, e.g. 2.5 mg salbutamol qds/prn
6. **CPAP:** Very low threshold for starting; some centres prefer CPAP > O_2 alone to help prevent atelectasis (even with relatively $\leftrightarrow PO_2$). CPAP may be easier to tolerate than chest physiotherapy with severe chest pain

7. **Chest physiotherapy:** Helps avoid atelectasis
8. **Thromboprophylaxis:** E.g. 40 mg enoxaparin od sc (if no contraindications)
9. **Blood transfusion:** Aim to ↓HbS and ↑ oxygenation. Only use if patient is anaemic: aim for Hb = 100 g/L. ☠ Hb ≥ 110 g/L may ↑viscosity and exacerbate sickling (an exchange transfusion preferable) ☠
10. **Exchange blood transfusion:** Discuss with haematology. Patient's blood is slowly removed and replaced with donor blood. Aim to ↓HbS < 20%
11. **HDU/ITU:** Admit to HDU/ITU where appropriate

UPPER AIRWAY OBSTRUCTION

☠ Life-threatening and requires prompt management! ☠ May occur **acutely** (e.g. foreign body) or **gradually** (e.g. tumour; sudden deterioration possible, e.g. sputum retention, Box 5.16.1). **Partial obstruction** → stridor or snoring; but **complete obstruction** → distress, paradoxical respiration, cyanosis and cardiorespiratory arrest.

5.16.1 Important causes of upper airway obstruction

- ↓GCS; unable to protect airway if < 8 (any cause)
- Obstruction by vomitus, blood, sputum or foreign body
- Epiglottitis
- Laryngeal oedema 2° to burns, inflammation or infection
- Anaphylaxis
- Internal obstruction or external compression by laryngeal or tracheal tumour/lymphadenopathy
- Angioedema (e.g. allergic, ACE inhibitors or hereditary)
- Bronchial oedema and bronchospasm (below level of larynx)
- Vocal cord paralysis
- Tracheal stenosis (e.g. post-intubation or tracheostomy)

IMMEDIATE MANAGEMENT

If cardiac or respiratory arrest → follow BLS/ALS immediately
(inside cover)
Always request senior anaesthetic help immediately!

Immediate priority: Avoid respiratory arrest by securing airway
using the following measures (as appropriate):

1. **Head tilt-chin lift** or **jaw-thrust** → if obstruction relieved (i.e.
   stridor stops and normal respiration pattern resumes) then insert
   oropharyngeal (Guedel) or **nasopharyngeal airway**
2. Visually inspect oropharynx and remove any obvious
   obstruction with a **finger sweep**
3. Use **Heimlich manoeuvre** if choking (firm and rapid upwards
   pressure applied beneath the diaphragm)
4. Use **suction** to remove any upper airway secretions
5. Attempt to remove any foreign body under direct vision using a
   laryngoscope and **McGill's forceps**
6. **Intubation** if required
7. **Cricothyroidotomy** (e.g. if unable to ventilate after intubation)

Definitive Rx depends on the underlying cause, e.g. surgery or
rigid bronchoscopy ± laser ± stenting for occlusions 2° to tumour.

ADDITIONAL HELPFUL MEASURES
FOR PARTIAL OBSTRUCTION

Heliox: Useful interim measure in partial obstruction 2° to
tumours. Helium and O_2 gas mixture (e.g. 80:20 or 70:30). Helium
has ↓ density, which improves airflow and work of breathing.
Immediately effective. Allows time to plan more definitive
treatment.

Nebulised adrenaline: Temporary measure. Most effective
in laryngeal oedema. Use 1 mL of 1:1000 with 4 mL of sodium
chloride 0.9%.

Reference Information

DOI: 10.1201/9781315151816-6

ARTERIAL BLOOD GAS INTERPRETATION

Arterial blood gases can help determine:

1. Oxygenation (PaO_2 > 7 kPa is adequate)
2. VQ mismatch (alveolar-arterial gradient; A-a O_2)
3. Alveolar ventilation ($PaCO_2$ > 6 kPa = hypoventilation; $PaCO_2$ < 4.7 kPa = hyperventilation)
4. Acid-base balance

NORMAL VALUES

pH	7.35–7.45
PaO_2	> 10.6 kPa*
$PaCO_2$	4.7–6 kPa
HCO_3^-	24–30 mmol/L
Lactate	0.5–2.2 mmol/L
Base Excess	± 2 mmol/L

* Inspiring room air at sea level.
< 10.6 kPa can be normal in elderly patients.
> 10.6 kPa is expected with supplemental O_2 (A-a gradient discussed hereunder).

ALVEOLAR-ARTERIAL GRADIENT (A-a O_2)

A measure of the difference between alveolar (A) O_2 and arterial (a) O_2.
↑ A-a gradient indicates VQ mismatch or shunting. Calculated using:

$$A - a\ O_2 = \text{Inspired } PO_2^* - \left(\text{arterial } PaO_2 + \frac{\text{arterial } PaCO_2}{0.8^{**}} \right)$$

Normal A-a O_2 = 1–2 kPa (*or* 2–3 kPa if elderly)

---

* Inspired PO_2 = FiO_2 (%) × (atmospheric pressure – water pressure)
   Example for patient inspiring 28% oxygen = 0.28 × (100 – 7) = 26 kPa.
** Respiratory quotient.

Worked example:

A 24-year-old male who is breathless on 24% oxygen. ABG: PaO_2 10.5 kPa and $PaCO_2$ 5 kPa.

Inspired $PO_2 = 0.24 \times (100 - 7) = 22.3$ kPa

$$A - a\ O_2 = 22.3 - \left(10.5 + \frac{5}{0.8}\right) = 5.6\ kPa$$

> 2 kPa, therefore patient has VQ mismatch

ACID-BASE BALANCE

This can be determined by plotting ABG results on the acid-base nomogram or alternatively using Table 6.1.

Anion gap

$[(Na^+ + K^+) - (Cl^- + HCO_3^-)]$ helps differentiate the cause of metabolic acidosis by calculating the presence of unmeasured

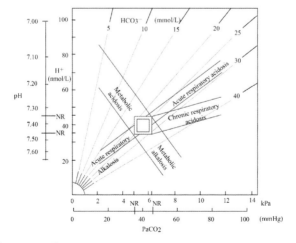

Figure 6.1 Acid-Base Nomogram.

Table 6.1 Determining the likely acid-base disorder from the pH, PaCO$_2$ and HCO$_3$

pH	PaCO$_2$	HCO$_3$	Acid-base disorder
↓	N	↓	**Primary metabolic acidosis**
↓	↓	↓	Metabolic acidosis with respiratory compensation
↓	↑	N	**Primary respiratory acidosis**
↓	↑	↑	Respiratory acidosis with renal compensation
↓	↑	↓	**Mixed metabolic and respiratory acidosis**
↑	↓	N	**Primary respiratory alkalosis**
↑	↓	↓	Respiratory alkalosis with renal compensation
↑	N	↑	**Primary metabolic alkalosis**
↑	↑	↑	Metabolic alkalosis with respiratory compensation
↑	↓	↑	**Mixed metabolic and respiratory alkalosis**

Note: Respiratory compensation occurs rapidly by changes in PaCO$_2$. Renal compensation occurs more slowly by changes in HCO$_3$. N, normal.

anions. It is a measure of 'fixed' or organic acids, e.g. phosphate, ketones and lactate. Normal range = 8–16 mmol/L.

Metabolic acidosis with normal anion gap, i.e. loss of HCO$_3^-$ or ingestion of H$^+$ (Cl$^-$ is retained):

1. Renal tubular acidosis
2. Diarrhoea
3. Acetazolamide
4. Addison's disease
5. Pancreatic fistulae
6. Ammonium chloride ingestion

Metabolic acidosis with ↑ anion gap, i.e. ingestion or ↑production of fixed/organic acids:

1. Lactic acidosis
2. ↑Uric acid (renal failure)
3. Ketoacidosis (diabetes, starvation or alcohol)
4. Salicylates, biguanides (metformin), ethylene glycol (antifreeze) or methanol ingestion

LUNG FUNCTION INTERPRETATION

SPIROMETRY

Plot of volume (y) against time (x) from a maximal forced
expiratory manoeuvre (Figure 6.2). The expiratory limb of the
flow-volume loop is also usually provided with standard electronic
spirometers and the same manoeuvre (discussed hereunder).

Three measures:

1. FEV_1 (<u>F</u>orced <u>E</u>xpiratory <u>V</u>olume in <u>1</u> second)
2. FVC (<u>F</u>orced <u>V</u>ital <u>C</u>apacity)
3. FEV_1/FVC ratio (ratio of above two measures)

FEV_1 and FVC are both provided as raw values (*litres*) and
corrected for age, sex, height and ethnic origin (% *predicted*).
FEV_1/FVC ratio is self-normalising.

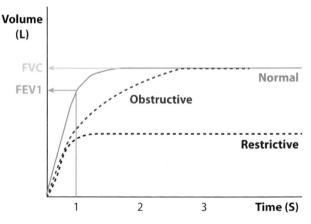

Figure 6.2 Spirometry (normal, obstructive and restrictive patterns).

Two major spirometry abnormalities (Box 6.2.1):

1. **Airflow obstruction** (e.g. COPD):
   - ↓FEV_1 *with* FEV_1/FVC **ratio < 0.7 (or 70%)**, i.e. the FVC is unaffected
2. **Restrictive** (e.g. ILD):
   - ↓FVC *with* FEV_1/FVC **ratio > 0.7 (or 70%; normal)**
   - ↓ in both lung volumes (FEV_1 & FVC) 4 FEV_1/FVC ratio always maintained[1]

6.2.1 Spirometry – Top Tips

- Always repeat the manoeuvre three times and record 'best' result
- Wide range of normality; therefore, serial measurements more helpful than 'one-off'
- Perform standing (with chair behind patient, as may become dizzy or pass out)
- Use a nose clip (if available)
- Keep patient blowing until a 'true' FVC is obtained (i.e. flat line or until 5 sec). This is important with airflow obstruction, where an underestimated FVC can bring the FEV_1/FVC ratio to within the normal range

In severe emphysema, loss of airway elasticity causes the airways to collapse during forced expiratory manoeuvres ('dynamic compression'). Better FEV_1 and FVC values can be obtained by asking the patient to repeat spirometry using a submaximal effort.

---

[1] Occasionally ↑FEV_1 with restrictive lung disease as airways are held open during forced expiration manoeuvre by fibrosed parenchymal attachments (i.e. ↓dynamic compression)→ ↑FEV_1/FVC ratio.

FLOW-VOLUME LOOP

Plot of expiratory (+) and inspiratory (−) flow (y) against lung volume (x) from a maximal forced expiratory manoeuvre followed immediately by a maximal and forced inspiratory manoeuvre (i.e. uninterrupted) (Figure 6.3).

Important measures include:

1. **PEFR** (**P**eak **E**xpiratory **F**low **R**ate)[1]
2. **FEF** (**F**orced **E**xpiratory **F**low), i.e. $FEF_{25\%}$, $FEF_{50\%}$, $FEF_{75\%}$ and $FEF_{25-75\%}$[2]
3. **FIF** (**F**orced **I**nspiratory **F**low), i.e. $FIF_{25\%}$, $FIF_{50\%}$, $FIF_{75\%}$ and $FIF_{25-75\%}$[2]

Most commonly, flow-volume loops are used to help identify more subtle airway obstruction affecting the small airways (e.g. asthma or early COPD). Here, the FEV_1 can be relatively normal, but the expiratory limb is 'bowed' with ↓ PEFR and FEFs (Figure 6.3). Other important abnormalities are shown in Figure 6.4.

GAS TRANSFER (CO TRANSFER, TLCO, DLCO OR κCO)

Measures the lung's ability to transfer gas from the inhaled air into the red bloods cells circulating within the alveolar capillaries ('gas exchange'). Performed in lung function laboratory. More involved than simple spirometry and requires a Hb. Cannot always be obtained, esp with very SOB patients. **Procedure**: *gas mixture containing CO is inhaled and the patient holds their breath for 10 sec. The difference between the inhaled and exhaled CO content is calculated to provide a measure of the CO that has been lost to the red blood cells by alveolar diffusion. This is corrected*

---

[1] **PEFR** is essentially what a peak flow meter measures.

[2] **FEF** and **FIF** are given at discrete times, defined by what fraction of the FVC remains (usually 25%, 50% and 75%), i.e. **FEF25%, FEF50%, FEF75%** or **FEF25%, FEF50%, FEF75%**. Average flow rates are also provided (**FEF25–75%** or **FIF25–75%**). There is a wide range of normality (FEF < 50% predicted is considered abnormal). All values are provided raw (L/sec) and corrected for age, sex, height and ethnic origin (**% predicted**).

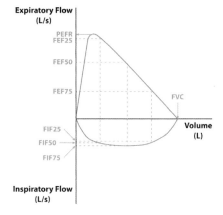

Figure 6.3 Flow-volume loop.

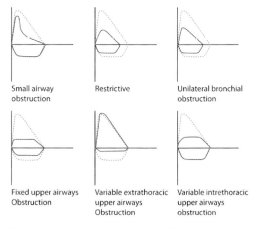

| Small airway obstruction | Restrictive | Unilateral bronchial obstruction |
| Fixed upper airways Obstruction | Variable extrathoracic upper airways Obstruction | Variable intrethoracic upper airways obstruction |

Figure 6.4 Important flow-volume loop abnormalities.

for the [Hb] as $\downarrow Hb \rightarrow CO$ *transfer.* **NB: tobacco** smoke contains CO and recent cigarette smoking can therefore affect results.

Two important measures:

1. **TLCO** (total amount of transferred CO; also **DLCO**)
2. **kCO** (TLCO ÷ total lung volume (discussed hereunder), i.e. gas transfer corrected for lung volume)

Abnormalities:

1. $\downarrow\downarrow$TLCO and $\downarrow\downarrow$kCO with emphysema (alveolar destruction)[1]
2. $\downarrow$TLCO and $\downarrow$kCO with ILD (thickened alveolar-capillary membrane)[1]
3. $\uparrow$kCO with profuse alveolar haemorrhage (e.g. Goodpasture's)[2]

BODY PLETHYSMOGRAPHY

Used to calculate lung volumes and is based on the principle of Boyle's law (i.e. pressure and volume are inversely proportional). **Procedure:** *patient sits in an airtight cabinet (closed and of known volume) resembling a telephone box. The patient breathes through a shuttered mouthpiece connected to the outside. Pressure Δs are measured by sensors in both the box and at the mouthpiece as the patient 'compresses' or 'rarefies' (expands) the air in their chest by exhaling or inhaling against the closed shutter respectively.* Lung volumes can then be calculated using pressure Δ as they are related to the volume of air being compressed or rarefied. Figure 6.5 shows how these values are influenced with disease.

Fractional exhaled nitric oxide (FeNO)

Higher than normal levels of NO are released by activated cells during inflammation, esp eosinophilic inflammation. FeNo measurements can

---

[1] Other conditions also $\downarrow$TLCO/kCO such as LVF or pulmonary hypertension.
[2] Blood (Hb) within the alveoli take up CO to 'falsely' $\uparrow$ kCO.

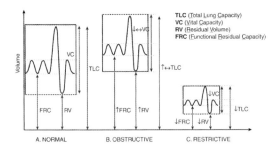

Figure 6.5 Lung volumes for normal, obstructive (e.g. COPD) and restrictive (e.g. ILD) lung conditions.

therefore provide an assessment of conditions such as asthma. Bedside, FeNO is now available (e.g. NIOX®) and can help in the diagnosis of asthma and guide in its treatment (Figure 6.6).

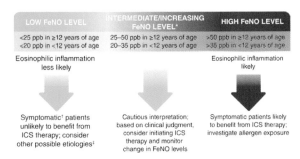

Figure 6.6 FeNo in the diagnosis and management of asthma. ICS = inhaled corticosteroid. (Adapted from http://www.niox.com/en-US/feno-asthma/interpreting-feno/.)

* Increasing is defined as an increase > 10 ppb from last measurement.
† Chronic cough and/or wheeze and/or shortness of breath for > 6 weeks.
‡ For example, rhinosinusitis, bronchiectasis, primary ciliary dyskinesia, anxiety-hyperventilation, cardiac disease, gastroesophageal reflux disease or vocal cord dysfunction.

NOTIFIABLE DISEASES AND CAUSATIVE ORGANISMS

Registered medical practitioners have a statutory duty to notify the 'proper officer' at the Local Council or local health protection team of suspected cases of certain infectious diseases. Advice can be found at: https://www.gov.uk/notifiable-diseases-and-causative-organisms-how-to-report.

A notification form should be completed immediately and sent within 3 days. Laboratory confirmation is NOT required. Urgent cases* require verbal notification within 24 h. All information is passed to Public Health England.

Diseases notifiable under the Health Protection (Notification) Regulations 2010 (*urgent):

- Acute encephalitis
- Acute infectious hepatitis*
- Acute meningitis*
- Acute poliomyelitis*
- Anthrax*
- Botulism*
- Brucellosis (*if UK-acquired)
- Cholera*
- Diphtheria*
- Enteric fever* (typhoid or paratyphoid fever)
- Food poisoning (*if clusters or outbreaks)
- Haemolytic uraemic syndrome*
- Infectious bloody diarrhoea*
- Invasive group A streptococcal disease*
- Legionnaires' disease*
- Leprosy
- Malaria
- Measles*
- Meningococcal septicaemia*
- Mumps
- Plague*
- Rabies*

- Rubella
- Severe Acute Respiratory Syndrome (SARS)*
- Scarlet fever
- Smallpox*
- Tetanus (*if associated with injected drug use)
- Tuberculosis (*if healthcare worker, cluster or MDR-TB)
- Typhus
- Viral haemorrhagic fever*
- Whooping cough (*if during acute phase)
- Yellow fever (*if UK-acquired)
- Report other diseases ('other significant disease') or contamination ('relevant contamination'), which may present significant risk to human health

Causative agents notifiable under the Health Protection (Notification) Regulations 2010:

- *Bacillus anthracis**
- *Bacillus cereus* (only if associated with food poisoning)
- *Bordetella pertussis**
- *Borrelia* spp.
- *Brucella* spp (*if UK-acquired)
- *Burkholderia mallei**
- *Burkholderia pseudomallei**
- *Campylobacter* spp.
- Chikungunya virus
- *Chlamydophila psittaci**
- *Clostridium botulinum**
- *Clostridium perfringens* (only if associated with food poisoning)
- *Clostridium tetani*
- *Corynebacterium diphtheria**
- *Corynebacterium ulcerans**
- *Coxiella burnetii* (*if acute phase or known cluster)
- Crimean-Congo haemorrhagic fever virus*
- *Cryptosporidium* spp. (*if known cluster, food-handler or evidence of ↑above expected numbers)
- Dengue virus (*if UK-acquired)

- Ebola virus*
- *Entamoeba histolytica*
- *Francisella tularensis**
- *Giardia lamblia* (*if known cluster, food-handler or evidence of ↑above expected numbers)
- Guanarito virus*
- *Haemophilus influenzae* (*if invasive)
- Hanta virus (*if UK-acquired)
- Hepatitis A, B, C, delta, and E viruses (*if acute case or chronic case that might represent a risk to others, e.g. healthcare worker)
- Influenza virus (*if new subtype, cluster or closed community, e.g. nursing home)
- Junin virus*
- Kyasanur Forest disease virus*
- Lassa virus*
- *Legionella* spp.*
- *Leptospira interrogans*
- *Listeria monocytogenes**
- Machupo virus*
- Marburg virus*
- Measles virus*
- Mumps virus
- Mycobacterium tuberculosis complex (*if healthcare worker, cluster or multi-drug resistance)
- *Neisseria meningitidis**
- Omsk haemorrhagic fever virus*
- *Plasmodium falciparum, vivax, ovale, malariae, knowlesi* (*if UK-acquired)
- Polio virus (wild or vaccine types)*
- Rabies virus (classical rabies and rabies-related lyssaviruses)*
- *Rickettsia* spp. (*if UK-acquired)
- Rift Valley fever virus*
- Rubella virus
- Sabia virus*
- *Salmonella* spp. (*if *S. typhi*, *S. paratyphi*, outbreak, food-handler or closed community, e.g. nursing home)

- SARS coronavirus*
- *Shigella* spp.*
- *Streptococcus pneumoniae* (only if invasive)
- *Streptococcus pyogenes* (only if invasive)*
- Varicella zoster virus
- Variola virus*
- Verocytotoxigenic *Escherichia coli* (including *E. coli* O157)*
- *Vibrio cholera**
- West Nile Virus (*if UK-acquired)
- Yellow fever virus (*if UK-acquired)
- *Yersinia pestis**

DRUG-INDUCED RESPIRATORY DISEASE

Many drugs are toxic to the lungs. Excellent aid at http://www.pneumotox.com/ (Dept of Pulmonary and Intensive Care, University Hospital, Dijon, France).

INDEX

Note: Locators in *italics* represent figures and **bold** indicate tables in the text.